A Legacy of Lessons Learned:

LANDSTUHL REGIONAL MEDICAL CENTER

DURING WARTIME

2001–2014

For sale by the Superintendent of Documents, U.S. Government Publishing Office
Internet: bookstore.gpo.gov   Phone: toll free (866) 512-1800;   DC area (202) 512-1800
Fax: (202) 512-2104 Mail: Stop IDCC, Washington, DC 20402-0001

ISBN 978-0-16-093504-6

A Legacy of Lessons Learned:

LANDSTUHL REGIONAL MEDICAL CENTER
DURING WARTIME
2001–2014

KAREN HENNESSY, RN, MS, CPNP

BORDEN INSTITUTE

US ARMY MEDICAL DEPARTMENT CENTER AND SCHOOL
HEALTH READINESS CENTER OF EXCELLENCE

FORT SAM HOUSTON, TEXAS

JOHN H. GARR, MD, MSE, FACEP | COLONEL, MC, US ARMY
Director and Editor in Chief, Borden Institute

JOAN REDDING
Senior Production Editor

VIVIAN MASON
Volume Editor

CHRISTINE GAMBOA, MS, MBA
Creative Director & Production Manager, Fineline Graphics, LLC

The opinions or assertions contained herein are the personal views of the author and are not to be construed as doctrine of the Department of the Army or the Department of Defense. Use of trade or brand names in this publication does not imply endorsement by the Department of Defense.

Published by the
OFFICE OF THE SURGEON GENERAL
BORDEN INSTITUTE
US ARMY MEDICAL DEPARTMENT CENTER AND SCHOOL
HEALTH READINESS CENTER OF EXCELLENCE
Fort Sam Houston, Texas
2016

Library of Congress Cataloging-in-Publication Data

Names: Hennessy, Karen, 1962- author. | Borden Institute (U.S.), issuing body.
Title: Legacy of lessons learned : Landstuhl Regional Medical Center during wartime, 2001-2014 / Karen Hennessy.
Description: Fort Sam Houston, Texas : Borden Institute, US Army Medical Department Center and School Health Readiness Center of Excellence, 2016. | Includes bibliographical references and index.
Identifiers: LCCN 2016039282
Subjects: | MESH: Landstuhl Regional Medical Center. | Hospitals, Military--history | Trauma Centers--history | Military Medicine--history | Afghan Campaign 2001- | Iraq War, 2003-2011 | Germany | United States
Classification: LCC RA989.G3 | NLM WX 28 GG4 | DDC 362.110943/43--dc23 LC record available at https://lccn.loc.gov/2016039282

PRINTED IN THE UNITED STATES OF AMERICA
23, 22, 21, 20, 19, 18, 17, 16   5 4 3 2 1

DEDICATION
WE DEDICATE THIS BOOK
TO THE REMARKABLE INDIVIDUALS WHO WORKED AT
LANDSTUHL REGIONAL MEDICAL CENTER
AND EPITOMIZED THE HOSPITAL'S MOTTO OF
"SELFLESS SERVICE"
DURING THIS CHALLENGING WARTIME PERIOD;
AND TO THE THOUSANDS OF
WOUNDED WARRIORS
WHO WERE TREATED AT
LANDSTUHL REGIONAL MEDICAL CENTER.
YOUR STRENGTH, COURAGE, RESILIENCY, AND SERVICE
TO YOUR COUNTRY HAVE BEEN AN
INSPIRATION TO A GENERATION OF AMERICANS.

Contents

Contributors

Executive Editors
Daniel E. Banks, MD, MS, MACP, LTC (Retired), MC, US Army
Timothy K. Jones, DDS, COL (Retired), DC, US Army

Greg Beilman, MD, COL, US Army Reserve, Trauma/Critical Care Surgeon
William Branch, Lt Col, US Marine Corps, Detachment Officer in Charge,
    Wounded Warrior Battalion East
Weyman Cannington, LTC, US Army, Chief, Patient Administration Division
Brenda Corrunker, Lt Col, US Air Force, Liaison Officer
Jane Darigo, RN, Outpatient Nurse Case Manager
Warren Dorlac, MD, COL, US Air Force, Medical Director, Trauma/
    Critical Care Unit; Director, C-STARS
Ray Fang, MD, Lt Col, US Air Force, Trauma/Critical Care Surgeon;
    Director, C-STARS
Joshua Forbess, SSG, US Army, Wounded Warrior Resiliency Program
Jeffrey B. Frazier, Deputy Chief, Patient Administration Division
Charles Frizzell, CMSgt, US Air Force, Liaison Officer
Philip Gilbert, MSgt, US Air Force, Liaison Officer
Kathryn Gillespie, RN, Chief Inpatient Nurse Case Manager
Robert Hinkel, Director, Laboratory Services
Darren Kasai, LT, US Army, Senior Noncommissioned
    Officer in Charge, DWMMC
Kevin Kirkpatrick, SSG, US Army, HMF (FMF) Liaison Officer
Kevin Kumlien, CDR, US Navy Reserve, Intensive Care Unit Nurse
Jeffrey Lawrence, SFC, US Army, Medical Transient Detachment

Foreword

For over 25 years, Landstuhl Regional Medical Center (LRMC) has served as a model of "selfless service," stepping up to the demands of a suddenly increased rate of traumatically injured service members arriving from the battlefield. From Operations Desert Storm/Desert Shield; through the attacks in Somalia, the Khobar Towers, and USS *Cole*; to the recent conflicts in Afghanistan and Iraq, LRMC has stood at the forefront of military healthcare, receiving our Nation's and our partners' wounded and ill from battlefields and contingencies across multiple theaters. From a community hospital providing routine healthcare delivery to personnel stationed in Europe and their families before 9/11, LRMC transitioned into a Level 1, triservice, integrated trauma center, providing lifesaving care to tens of thousands of evacuated service members, in addition to handling all the associated needs of these patients, from payroll assistance to chaplain services, service and unit liaison support, and veteran service organization support, as well as delivering ongoing healthcare to beneficiaries across Europe, Africa, and Asia.

The goal of this text is to share the lessons learned by LRMC staff in converting from a peacetime to wartime footing, serving as a guide for US military hospitals in similar situations in the future. The innovations and solutions planned and implemented so successfully by LRMC staff will assist future military medical and line leaders in maintaining the highest quality of healthcare services for future generations of our service men and women in combat, improving upon the historically high survival rates seen in these conflicts.

BRIAN C LEIN
MAJOR GENERAL
Staff Surgeon, 2nd General Hospital and LRMC, 1993–1996
Commander, Landstuhl Regional Medical Center, 2007–2009

Fort Detrick, Maryland
July 2016

Acknowledgments

A special thank you to Commander Lisa Lewis, US Navy Reserve, Outpatient Nurse Case Manager, our point of contact at Landstuhl Regional Medical Center (LRMC). Her efficiency, dedication, and commitment to this project made this book possible. We also thank her commanding officer, Captain Laurie Wesely, US Navy, who supported this book both at LRMC and upon her return home.

We thank Charles Roberts and Marie Shaw of LRMC's Public Affairs Office for reviewing the manuscript and providing photos, resources, and contributors. The legacy of lessons learned addressed in this book spanned a period of more than a dozen years, and their long service at LRMC proved invaluable to understanding the progression and growth of this unique medical facility.

We are grateful to all of the individuals from designated units at LRMC who contributed to each chapter's content by sharing their knowledge and experience from various periods of service. We also thank those individuals we interviewed who gave us hours of their time, providing valuable information and perspective through their personal stories and experiences: Warren Dorlac, Joshua Forbess, Robert Hinkel, Kevin Kirkpatrick, Kevin Kumlien, Kathleen Martin, Mary Norgaard, Shelley Ohlendorf, Pam Patnode, Ronald Pettigrew, Carol Weingarten, Michael Weingarten, and David Zonies. We are indebted to Colonel Martha K. Lenhart for her vision, persistence, and enthusiasm for this project. We thank Lieutenant Colonel (Retired) Daniel Banks and Colonel (Retired) Timothy Jones of Borden Institute for their assistance in reviewing and editing the manuscript.

Introduction

The quiet, quaint village of Landstuhl, Germany, is located in the Rheinland-Pfalz province, about 90 miles southwest of Frankfurt, close to the French border. Tucked comfortably in a small valley, the village is surrounded on three sides by notably sized hills. Locals and visitors enjoy the walk to the restaurants and shops that reflect the flavors of this community, as well as the view of Burg Nanstein, a 15th century castle overlooking the entire village. At the bottom of one of these hills is a long, steep driveway that has earned the nickname "Cardiac Hill." No one would know that beyond the thick forest of trees on either side of that driveway is an American military base with a compelling story and a hospital that has saved thousands of lives.

History of Landstuhl Regional Medical Center

The Landstuhl area has a rich history tracing to Celtic and Roman times. In 1796, the area was taken over by the French and later became part of the French Empire under Napoleon Bonaparte. After Waterloo, Landstuhl became part of the Kingdom of Bavaria. After Germany was formed in the late 19th century, breweries and factories brought wealth to the area. Landstuhl also became known as a spa resort, attracting patients suffering from arthritis and other diseases.

German soldiers who died in World War I were buried in a small cemetery near the 13th century chapel in downtown Landstuhl. In early 1938, construction of the Hitlerjugend Schule (Hitler Youth School) began on one of the hilltops, the site that later became home to Landstuhl Regional Medical Center. Some of the buildings from the Youth School are still on the military post today. On March 19, 1945, US troops entered Landstuhl. The US Army has maintained a hospital presence in the town of Landstuhl since November 28, 1951, when the 320th General Hospital took over operational control from an existing German military hospital. Construction soon began on a new facility, which admitted the first 375 patients on March 9, 1953.

The following year, the facility was renamed the 2nd General Hospital. Its facilities expanded throughout the Cold War era. The hospital not only provided healthcare within the European theater, but also played an integral role in patient care during high profile terrorist incidents and disasters: for example, caring for US Marines injured during the aborted 1980 rescue attempt of American hostages in Iran and caring for those injured in the 1983 bombing of the US Marine Corps barracks in Beirut, Lebanon. Soldiers injured during the 1986 LaBelle Discothèque bombing in Berlin and the 500 casualties of the 1988 Ramstein Air Show disaster were also treated at the hospital in Landstuhl. From August 1990 through March 1991, more than 4,000 service members injured during Operation Desert Shield and Operation Desert Storm and more than 800 military personnel deployed to Somalia between 1992 and 1994 were evacuated and treated at the 2nd General Hospital.

In 1994, the hospital was renamed the Landstuhl Army Medical Center, and it continued to serve as the primary medical center for casualties of US operations within Europe, southwest Asia, and the Middle East. In August 1998, the hospital treated American and Kenyan victims of the US Embassy bombing in Nairobi, supported the repatriation of three American prisoners of war in 1999, and treated the sailors injured in the USS Cole bombing. In November 2003, the hospital was renamed Landstuhl Regional Medical Center (LRMC), and subsequently included personnel from all branches of the military. In addition to providing specialty care to patients in the Kaiserslautern area, LRMC became the evacuation platform for casualties of US overseas contingency operations in the European, African, and Central commands.

LRMC is the only US Role 4 medical treatment facility outside the United States and, from 2011 to 2014, it was the military's only Level I trauma center overseas. Since 2003, every wounded warrior from Afghanistan and Iraq has come to LRMC to receive care. More than 90,000 sick and injured patients from Operation Enduring Freedom, Operation Iraqi Freedom, and Operation New Dawn have been treated at LRMC to date.

The Evolution of a World-Class Medical Facility

The events of September 11, 2001 forever changed our nation. They also changed the operational landscape of LRMC. As the largest US military healthcare facility in Europe, LRMC found itself in a unique position as the common link between Central Command and continental US medical facilities. Because of its location, LRMC became a pivotal strategic evacuation center across a spectrum of conflict stretching over thousands of miles and three continents. LRMC could no longer be seen as a community hospital delivering routine medical care to European service members and their families; the Global War on Terrorism transformed it into a world-class trauma center addressing the needs of seriously ill and injured wounded warriors and saving thousands of lives.

The first post-9/11 casualty arrived at LRMC in October 2001. Over the next year, approximately 25,000 troops were sent to Afghanistan, and by December 2002, the hospital was feeling the impact of increased patient volume. It became clear that additional administrative and clinical assistance was needed to support this effort. Tracking patients and medical management were not feasible with its previous resources. Some of the units and programs described in this book—such as the Deployed Warrior Medical Management Center, the Medical Transient Detachment, and the Wounded Warrior Finance Office—did not previously exist. In 2003, LRMC requested and received 400 Army and 200 Air Force reserve personnel to augment the existing Table of Distribution and Allowances staff. Additional staff came from the Navy in 2006.

Challenges continued to arise at LRMC despite the additional staffing. The survival rate of soldiers injured in combat had significantly increased due to improvements in protective body armor, advances in trauma care, and knowledge gained by medical personnel in the prehospital far-forward environment. However, the type of warfare engaged in by combatants, the types of injuries sustained, the duration of deployments, the number of redeployments, and the short down time between deployments made these wars fundamentally different. New and additional medical and surgical specialists were required to adequately evaluate and treat the arriving wounded warriors. Innovations born of these challenges became part of the valuable lessons learned at LRMC. The synergistic relationship between military and civilian trauma care proved to be an essential asset. Fellowship-trained trauma surgeons advocated for tools such as trauma registries, performance improvement processes, and clinical practice guidelines. The growing awareness of the significant impact of traumatic brain injuries (TBIs) led to the development of mandatory TBI screening for all patients evacuated to LRMC. The development of a TBI program at LRMC benefited all patients who presented at LRMC with head injuries and cognitive symptoms. The initiation of the Critical Care Air Transport Team was instrumental in significantly reducing patient morbidities and mortalities. The success of this "flying hospital" program continues to have far-reaching impact for both military and peacetime missions.

The medical staff at LRMC performed just about every surgery possible from head to foot, from sports injuries to injuries from improvised explosive devices. LRMC staff treated soldiers with burns, tumors, diabetes, depression, and posttraumatic stress disorder. Before 2001, LRMC would have considered admitting 30 to 40 patients in a day as a mass casualty event. Instead, this pace became the new norm, and staff adapted accordingly. This was accomplished while LRMC remained committed to the mission of treating retirees, local service members, and their families stationed in Europe. Since January 2004, 21% of patients evacuated to LRMC have suffered from battle injuries, whereas the remainder was disease- or nonbattle injury-related. Remarkably, more than 20% of wounded warriors who were treated at LRMC returned to duty. This rate equates to more than 19 battalions that LRMC was instrumental in keeping in the fight.

People are the lifeline of any organization, and this fact was never exemplified more clearly than at "Larmcy," the affectionate nickname given to LRMC. The factors that remained consistent throughout this period of war were the unwavering dedication, commitment to excellence, and humanitarian effort represented in the hospital's motto of "selfless service." These values were seen in every corner and in every hallway of LRMC, from administrative staff, to the Wounded Warrior Finance Office, to liaison officers, chaplains, laboratory services, clinicians, and volunteers. Although a sick and wounded soldier may only have spent 24 to 72 hours at LRMC, these patients humbled, inspired, and motivated an entire hospital community whose relentless purpose centered on doing whatever it took to save lives, diminish suffering, and offer comfort in any way possible.

LRMC continued to evolve to meet the needs of wounded warriors. For more than a decade of war, the lessons learned at LRMC were invaluable and ongoing. Capturing these lessons became a priority, and this book was written with the purpose of identifying and understanding the integral role of LRMC as a strategic evacuation center across the spectrum of conflict. These lessons not only contribute to the history of military medicine, but also serve as an essential resource should another military medical facility need to replicate LRMC's evolution.

The battlefield did not stop at the borders of Iraq and Afghanistan. C-17 cargo planes landing at Ramstein Air Base brought the war to Landstuhl, Germany, at all hours of the day and night. The extraordinary endeavor that went on daily in the last 13-plus years of conflict have validated and proven the vital role of LRMC as a world-class military medical center.

What is Success?

To laugh often and much;
to win the respect of intelligent people
and the affection of children.
To earn the appreciation of honest critics
and the betrayal of false friends;
To appreciate beauty,
To find the best in others;
To leave the world a bit better,
whether by a healthy child,
a garden patch, or a redeemed social condition;
To know even one life has breathed easier
because you have lived.
This is to have succeeded.[*]

*According to the Ralph Waldo Emerson Society and the English department of Texas A&M University (http://emerson-legacy.tamu.edu/Ephemera/Success.html), this poem, although often attributed to Emerson, was published as "What is Success?" by Bessie A. Stanley, in: Chapple JM, ed. *Heart Throbs*, Vol 2. Boston, MA: Chapple Publishing Company; 1911.

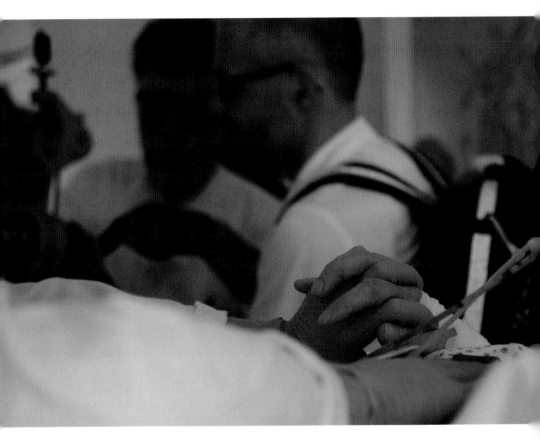

A nurse holds a patient's hand while being transferred to the
hospital, July 9, 2013, at Landstuhl Regional Medical Center,
Germany. An active-duty Air Force crew made history while flying
specialized medical teams, and their patient required medical
equipment never before used on board a Transatlantic mission.

CHAPTER ONE

A Soldier's Story

*Sometimes you are lucky enough in life to meet a person who profoundly
impacts you, someone who makes you want to be a better person, someone
who changes your life simply by the way that he has lived his. And when you
are privileged enough to hear his story, you recognize the extraordinary in his
ordinary; his day-to-day living, humbly going about his business with intent
and purpose despite the overwhelming obstacles he's faced.*

The mission statement for Fort Campbell, Kentucky, flows along the top of its website: *I will always place the mission first. I will never accept defeat. I will never quit. I will never leave a fallen comrade.* That is exactly the commitment Private Josh Forbess engrained in his soul when he joined the Army 2 days after his 18th birthday, a mere moment after he officially went from boy to man. This was a decision made to broaden his experiences from the small town in Illinois he had known all his life. The military career aptitude test targeted his innate mathematical and mechanical abilities, which were a perfect skill match for a Field Artilleryman: a soldier trained to fight on foot and attack the enemy in face-to-face combat. Athletic, with strong muscles, quick feet, and a sharp, keen mind, Josh Forbess was a natural for this position in the Army.

Two years later, at age 20, he was deployed for the first time. Both Bosnia and Kosovo were considered peacekeeping missions, but to a small-town young man, neither place looked anything but peaceful. This was his first exposure to a developing country: refugees in broken down half-way houses, skeletal limbs starving for food, listless eyes starving for hope, fear peering from the eyes of the young and old with no certainty for a safe day, much less a safe future. It was poverty and devastation to a degree he never knew possible. Forbess will tell you that there is a certain point in every man's life when he finds out who he really is. This was that experience. It "set him, grounded him," catalyzing his philosophy, his mind-set, his commitment to be the best he could be. That turning point to a new level of self-growth and self-awareness might have been one of the most important events in his life, an eerie foreshadowing to prepare the 20-year-old for an even greater challenge to come.

Fast forward to 2003. Life was good for 26-year-old Josh, now Sergeant (SGT) Forbess, who seemingly was on the fast track in his career. He loved the military, was engaged to be married, and his life had both personal and professional meaning. Josh deployed out of Fort Campbell to Iraq on March 8, 2003. Dates become particularly relevant to a person when one day or one timeframe separates your life from everything you know as normal to nothing ever being the same again.

The date he will never forget was November 15, 2003. Josh was conducting "Eyes Over Mosul," an aerial quick-reaction force mission providing surveillance support from the air to where ground disruption was stirring. One instant to the next became transforming that day: flying overhead in a UH60 Black Hawk utility helicopter, then the sound of an explosion, black smoke circling the air, and a life about to change forever. His memory of exact details is somewhat sketchy, and most of what he knows was told to him. An RPG (rocket-propelled grenade) hit another Black Hawk helicopter that was close by, but not part of their mission. That aircraft was transporting troops between bases. The second Black Hawk hit them midair, taking off their tail rotor (back wing). Both planes were spinning wildly out of control when another RPG exploded into their helicopter, slamming them onto the roof of a house. The second Black Hawk also crashed, hitting the side of a school. For Josh, it then went black.

That unforeseen, gut-wrenching ending to "Eyes Over Mosul" took the lives of 17 soldiers. All ten passengers in the second Black Hawk were killed, as were seven of the twelve 101st Airborne Division soldiers in Josh's aircraft. SGT Forbess was the most severely injured of the remaining survivors and the only one who could be pulled out from inside the wreckage. He was taken to a combat hospital in Mosul, then Baghdad, and from there flown to Landstuhl Regional Medical Center (LRMC) in Germany. After a CT (computed tomography) scan and emergency hand surgery, SGT Forbess was whisked back to the United States to Brooke Army Medical Center (BAMC) in San Antonio, Texas. From the moment of crash landing in Mosul to being wheeled into BAMC was a period of just 36 hours. He was still covered in soot. Josh Forbess has no memory of any of this.

There was nothing minor about any of his injuries. SGT Forbess had severe burns to his face, head, right shoulder, and right arm. Bones were broken in both of his hands. His lungs, drenched in black, looked like the inside of a coal mine. Josh developed pneumonia from severe smoke inhalation and had extensive lung damage. He was on a ventilator for 2 weeks and spent 2 months in the intensive care unit where he was placed in a medically induced coma. The burns took his ear and half of his nose.

January 11, 2004: another significant date. It was the first one Josh remembers after coming out of his coma. He recalls looking on a computer to actually see the date and then looking at the NFL schedule (the Packers played the Eagles that day). His life from November 15, 2003 up to this very point was a complete blank. The details of his life for those 8 weeks and the details of that fateful November day were then told to him. He remembers asking how many soldiers were lost and where his fiancée was.

And so began a long, painful, and heroic return to a life now drastically different from anything he had ever anticipated. Josh suffered extensive 3rd and 4th degree burns to 11% of his body, 7% to his face and head, and 4% to his right arm. His life became a series of reconstructive surgeries and skin engraftments, from eyelids to nose to ear to right arm. He recounts his complex medical history matter-of-factly, as if he had recovered from a minor car accident rather than a helicopter explosion. He has told his story so many times and will tell you he has mastered separating the facts from the emotion. He has, however, never lost his dry sense of humor. "They took my latissimus dorsi (broadest back muscle) and a skin flap from my right butt cheek to engraft my skull," Forbess states. "That makes me a REAL genuine butthead!"

Josh also states that he is not sure if it was the pain itself he remembers or the pain from the depression. "Mental pain is way harder than the physical," he states, once envisioning himself looking like the elephant man. Josh attributes his first step to acceptance to J. R. Martinez, a fellow infantryman from Fort Campbell who had been deployed to Iraq in February 2003. Two months later, Martinez was driving a High Mobility Multipurpose Wheeled Vehicle (or HMMWV—pronounced "Humvee") when its front tire hit an IED (improvised explosive device). He suffered smoke inhalation and severe burns and, like Josh, was evacuated to LRMC and then transferred to the Burn Center at BAMC. Josh recalls his first visit, when 20-year-old Martinez walked into his room, completely unfazed by scars, skin grafts, or disfigurement, his own included. Martinez announced, "I am who I am and the hell with everybody else." How cool was that? thought Forbess, who was awed by this strength, courage, and determination. Later that night, Josh picked up a mirror to look at his face for the first time. The journey to healing and self-acceptance, however, was long and painful, and Forbess admits that there were many dark hours. He was given a 30-day convalescence before officially being discharged from the Burn Center. He returned home to Illinois at that time. His demons followed. Anger, guilt, and sadness raged an ugly war within as he struggled daily with the fact that he lived and his comrades had died. He blamed himself for crawling out and leaving his men behind. It was not until months later that he learned the whole story of how he survived: that in fact he did not crawl out, but had to be pulled out from the wreckage.

Forbess spent $5,000 on alcohol during those 30 days trying desperately to numb the pain in any way possible. He was very clear on his purpose during that time. Alcohol gave him a means to drink himself into a dream world of being an uninjured soldier in the greatest division in the greatest Army in the world. In that dream, he is firing a Howitzer. It's fun, he's a natural; this is what he was trained to do. Josh awakened instead to a nightmare called reality. He continued drinking as a way to return to that dream.

He returned to BAMC and underwent a series of surgeries to rebuild his nose and ear. At some point in 2004, Josh had an epiphany. His group of guys would never want him living like this. He loved the military, and he refused to believe his career was over. His honesty is painstakingly real, as he also admitted to being *afraid* to leave the Army. It was the life he knew and where he felt most comfortable in his own skin.

SGT Forbess got his drinking under control and in 2004 returned to Fort Campbell, where he was assigned to administrative duty. Even though he was not firing a Howitzer as in his dreams, he was with his unit. It was like returning home to be with his family. In December 2004, he was promoted to Staff Sergeant (SSG) Forbess. He stayed at Fort Campbell until 2007, when the command team had an idea about how to better utilize his experiences. He was given an opportunity to work in the hospital at Fort Campbell, where they were setting up an Ombudsman program, an organization established by the Army in 2007 as a support service and resource augmentation for soldiers and their families. SSG Forbess would serve as a Wounded Warrior Advocate. Josh had been visiting soldiers in the hospital on his own time; he now had a formal title and position. This job turned out to be the stepping stone for his future position at LRMC. After 6 months, he became the Noncommissioned Officer in Charge at Fort Campbell's Soldier and Family Assistance Center (SFAC), where he supported warriors in transition and their families. In 2006, the Fort Campbell Fisher House opened, the home built on post for military families to reside in while a loved one was receiving medical treatment. Josh was a regular volunteer, leading wounded warrior meetings and sharing his story.

In August 2011, SSG Forbess was assigned to LRMC to continue his mission at the Wounded Warrior Resiliency Program. The title of this program was particularly relevant to Forbess, who sees resiliency as the master key in unlocking the healing process. His credibility is his Midas touch. Forbess feels it is important to talk about his own black days, which were every bit a part of his story as the work he does now. Nothing was more real than living that raw emotional pain. It gave him a unique and genuine launching pad to relate to other soldiers facing similar struggles. "No one can tell you what it feels like to be blown up except someone who has been blown up." No argument there, soldier!

He often relies on a Native American philosophy that helped him in his darkest hours: a belief that there is a 1-year grieving period that is necessary, and then it is time to let go and move forward. We cannot stay stuck in the past forever.

There is no formal protocol to his approach when he meets each wounded soldier. He knows that as soon as he walks in the room, they know "he has been there and back." His goal is to gain their trust. That is most important. He breaks the ice by just hanging out, telling jokes, and getting them to laugh. He will help transport them to various tests if needed. Josh might tell parts of his story, but more importantly, he wants them to tell theirs. SSG Forbess relies on instinct, experience, and "just being real" to assess whether soldiers are really spilling their pain or repressing it. "You have to talk about it," he tells them, "really talk about it, and not the kind of talking you do when you are out drinking with your buddies." It might take a while for someone to start opening up; once that happens, you never want to lose that emotional momentum, that moment of opportunity. SSG Forbess might be in a room for an hour, sometimes 5 or 6 hours, or sometimes a soldier wakes up and he is still there. Forbess stays until his work is done. The clear message he wants them to know is "My brother's got my back."

Josh reflects on his own experience, those first weeks and months when he came out of the coma. He is honest with his assessment. This was a new war. No one was really prepared to deal with the volume of patients, the complexity of injuries, or the degree of psychological ramifications for these wounded warriors. During the Vietnam conflict, most soldiers with the types of injuries he sustained would have died. This was 30 years later and an entirely different battlefield. Josh himself was the first surviving soldier with life-threatening burns who had experienced the loss of fellow soldiers. At the time, the psychology team did not really know how to help him. Josh does not blame anyone, nor is he angry. There was no instruction manual for this type of devastation. What he does painfully remember, however, is how alone and lost he felt digging himself inch by inch out of the grave of emotional hell. That is what he tries to prevent for every wounded warrior who comes his way. He does not want to see a new generation of disgruntled veterans. "These are my brothers and sisters," Josh states. "It is us taking care of us. No one is alone."

Healing is hard work. Healing takes time. There is no shortcut or bypass or escape. Josh lives with daily reminders of that fateful November day. He has TBI (traumatic brain injury), which has resulted in challenges with word associations and short-term memory loss. He has been told that he has PTSD (posttraumatic stress disorder). Scars, grafts, and broken bones have restricted the full range of mobility in his arm and hands. These are not the problems, however, Forbess chooses to focus on. Eight and a half years after the accident, Josh awoke one morning and felt totally at peace. He is grateful for what is good in his life: a job with purpose and a spouse who understood "in good times and in bad" long before those official wedding vows were spoken. Back in 2003, his 20-year-old fiancée never left his side. A nursing student at the time, she flew to be with him in the intensive care unit in San Antonio. An extraordinary young woman, she stood by him during those 30 dark days when he bathed his pain in alcohol, through dozens of surgeries, and through every twist and turn of his remarkable journey. Josh Forbess was married on September 3, 2005, and his wife works as a nurse at LRMC.

SSG Forbess feels it is essential to pass on lessons he has learned to future facilities and caretakers that may face a similar challenge, including the following:

- A caring hospital staff is essential.
- Be honest; truth is critical.
- Never assume that a patient "hears" what you are telling him or her the first time. Keep repeating and re-telling the information as if it is the first time the patient is hearing it. It may take multiple efforts before it all sinks in.
- The impact of sharing experiences cannot be underestimated. It is so valuable to both the patients and their families.
- The first step to healing others is to first start with healing yourself.

Not a day goes by that SSG Forbess does not think about his fallen comrades—those men that were his family. They are his lessons learned, his "raison d'être." It is in their memory that he had the courage to put one foot in front of the other and continue to live. Forbess recommits to his purpose daily:

- Never let their memories fade. As soon as they fade, they truly die.
- Always keep them smiling down on me.
- Keep their families proud.

On any given day at any given hour, soldiers, patients, and caregivers will be seen along the 3 miles of hallways at LRMC. SSG Josh Forbess has lived each one of these roles. He is the *soldier* who understands commitment to the mission, the *patient* who has lived the word "suffering," and the *caregiver* who practices putting patients first. It is what makes his perspective so valuable, his story so unique.

What is it about the resiliency of a human spirit that can reach down to the depths of unbearable despair, and somehow surface to face the world with unfathomable courage, integrity, and resolve? Josh Forbess faced unspeakable loss at every corner he took a breath: the death of men he called brothers, a dream career shattered in the debris of a helicopter wreckage, and a stranger staring back in the mirror. Diligent surgeons carefully worked to restructure and realign the face of SSG Josh Forbess, who was then tasked to diligently restructure and realign the architecture of his own life.

The following chapters in this book depict the development and implementation of various units and programs that grew out of sheer necessity to both save and rebuild lives. SSG Josh Forbess represents the epitome of what made LRMC one of the greatest lessons learned during this war.

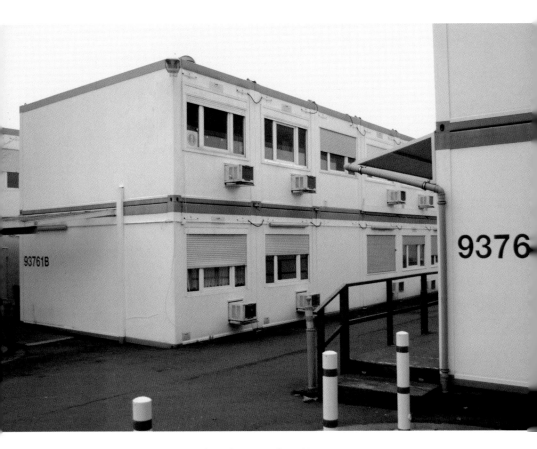

These unique two-story modular trailer units were adjacent to the hospital and home to the Deployed Warrior Medical Management Center.

CHAPTER TWO

Patient Administration Division and Deployed Warrior Medical Management Center

It is one thing to admit and discharge sick patients who live locally;
it is quite another when that same process now involves admitting
and discharging evacuated patients from thousands of miles away,
communicating with families thousands of miles away, and safeguarding
and accounting for funds and valuables of patients from all over the world.

Before any wounded warrior arrived at Landstuhl Regional Medical Center (LRMC), many wheels of the patient support system were already set in motion. Behind the scenes of direct patient care are hospital administrative services that address a multitude of necessary functions integral to the delivery of quality care. These essential services are particularly complex in the military during wartime as administrative responsibilities become more global. It is one thing to admit and discharge sick patients who live locally; it is quite another when that same process now involves admitting and discharging evacuated patients from thousands of miles away, communicating with families thousands of miles away, and safeguarding and accounting for funds and valuables of patients from all over the world. This complexity does not eliminate the other routine responsibilities of administrative services such as: ensuring HIPPA (Health Insurance Portability and Accountability Act) compliance and training, reporting medical data, documenting appropriated medical coding, and maintaining medical records for wounded warriors and local civilians needing medical care from birth to death and everything in between.[1]

The Patient Administration Division (PAD) at LRMC has always been a patient-centric service organization that carried out varied responsibilities on a daily basis. Through teamwork and collaboration, PAD's goal was to consistently provide professional, administrative support to clinical staff; ensure patient satisfaction; and sustain quality medical documentation. The PAD mission statement at LRMC is as follows:

> *A collaborative, well trained, and ready team that enables our clinical staff to provide safe, world-class healthcare for our patients to maximize their health and well-being through accurate medical documentation and quality patient administrative services.*[1]

The Deployed Warrior Medical Management Center (DWMMC) was a unique organization at LRMC that also played an integral role in providing medical and administrative management to US military service members evacuated from supported theaters. The DWMMC originally grew from the PAD Aeromedical Evacuation (PADAE) office. The center evolved from an internally LRMC-staffed entity into a triservice and civilian organization staffed through the global force management process and funded by the Overseas Contingency Operations (OCO) budget. The development of this comprehensive systems approach to casualty management facilitated patient evacuation and accountability during Operation Enduring Freedom (OEF) and Operation Iraqi Freedom (OIF). The DWMMC was responsible for tracking all patients being evacuated from the combatant commands and served as the permanent link between the combat theater and continental US (CONUS) medical facilities. This integral unit coordinated services across eight functional areas: (1) clinical management, (2) patient administration and logistical support for incoming patients, (3) healthcare delivery, (4) redeployment processing, (5) billeting and lodging, (6) case management, (7) financial and logistical support, and (8) outbound movement.[2]

The mission of the DWMMC is as follows:

> *To coordinate and facilitate triage, reception, medical management, and onward movement of wounded warriors from overseas contingency operations (OCO) in the US Central Command (CENTCOM), US Africa Command (AFRICOM), and US European Command (EUCOM) areas of responsibility (AORs).*[2]

BACKGROUND

The Evolution of Service: Patient Administration Division to the Deployed Warrior Medical Management Center

After the events of September 11, 2001, LRMC became the logical evacuation platform for personnel coming from the CENTCOM AOR (US Central Command area of responsibility) who needed sophisticated medical testing, specialty care appointments, short-term treatment, and inpatient care, due to its strategic location and medical capabilities. At that time, LRMC was not structured to handle such an increase in patient volume, which resulted in prolonged delays of outpatient treatment.

With the announcement that the United States would be sending 25,000 troops to Afghanistan (OEF) in 2001, LRMC began a series of meetings with personnel who were at LRMC during Operation Desert Shield/Operation Desert Storm (ODS/ODS). One of the lessons learned during that war was the importance of LRMC continuing its peacetime mission (ie, caring for local beneficiaries and other eligible patients), while also receiving and caring for wounded warriors from downrange. During ODS/ODS, LRMC had put its peacetime mission on hold and admitted 100% of patients arriving from theater. While admitting that all contingency patients solved problems in patient tracking and command and control, it turned out to be a huge problem for local beneficiaries who then had to rely solely on German hospitals for inpatient and specialty care. This proved to be a catastrophic financial issue for retirees over 65 years of age because, at that time, military insurance (CHAMPUS or Civilian Health and Medical Program of the Uniformed Services) paid for medical care at civilian facilities for all beneficiaries until they turned 65, after which they were no longer eligible for civilian care reimbursement. Free medical care could then only be obtained at a military medical facility. Many of those affected lost their life savings to pay for necessary medical treatment. LRMC did not want this situation to occur again during this war.

The chief and deputy chief of PAD discussed the needs of patients coming from theater. Based on experiences during ODS/ODS, as well as patients from the Balkans, Somalia, and the USS *Cole*, it was determined that the best approach would be to establish a separate unit specifically responsible for managing wounded warriors. The logical foundation for this new entity was the PADAE, with augmentation from other PAD personnel and hospital clinical staff.

PAD was divided into several sections, each with a different AOR. The PADAE was specifically responsible for processing requests for air evacuation to CONUS for patients needing more complex care elsewhere, or those needing continuous care at another medical facility. Prior to OEF the PADAE consisted of two junior enlisted personnel. Their mission was to enter patients into the TRANS-COM Regulating and Command & Control Evacuation System (TRAC2ES) who were referred by providers at LRMC to CONUS medical treatment facilities. Additionally, they produced travel orders for all patients departing LRMC for medical care in CONUS. They also tracked and provided support to patients from Kosovo and Bosnia. Patient tracking once consisted of a Microsoft Excel spreadsheet, which eventually developed into the Department of Defense (DoD) patient tracking system now known as the Theater Medical Data Store (TMDS).

In response to the new logistical and operational challenges that arose with OEF and OIF, various units or "cells" were developed in PAD. Each cell had its own unique set of tasks, but all tasks were interrelated. The need to streamline and improve patient movement prompted PAD to make a proposal to LRMC to establish a new unit that would provide logistic support to patients coming from the CENTCOM theater, including billeting, meals, clothing, and transportation. This new organization would also work closely with clinical staff on early notification and planning for receiving inbound patients. The traditional medical holding company was used as the model for the initial development of this organization. The new unit was approved in October 2001, coincident with the beginning of OEF. Daily meetings were held with PAD, nursing, and clinical staff members to review the inbound patient movement requests (PMRs) and make ward assignments.

A NEW UNIT EMERGES

From October 2001, when the unit was approved, until early 2003, the unit that was initially named the *Deployed Warrior Medical Care Center* was then changed to its current name and consisted of 10 personnel. With the buildup of troops for OIF and the arrival of 400 US Army reservists and 200 US Air Force reservists at LRMC, the DWMMC expanded to more than 100 personnel and came under the leadership of an Army Medical Corps lieutenant colonel and a Medical Service Corps captain.[1]

With the new command at the DWMMC, PAD then stepped back and provided a supporting role, while still continuing on with its original mission. The only exception was that the PADAE remained a part of the DWMMC, and continued to process orders and input TRAC2ES information for all patients (contingency and noncontingency) departing LRMC for further care elsewhere.[1] The DWMMC then assumed the following responsibilities:
- administrative: reporting and recording medical information in the computer before a patient arrives;
- air evacuation: monitoring departures from downrange to arrival at LRMC;
- case management: nursing coordination of outpatient care;
- mission teams;
- logistics: addressing essential patient needs from luggage handling to clothing to medical appointments;

- triage: assessing severity of the patient's condition from downrange to arrival;
- billeting;
- maintaining movement sections: tracking patient evacuation movement worldwide; and
- coordination: collaborating with other LRMC personnel, such as liaisons and chaplain services, for nonmedical needs.

By 2006, sourcing LRMC augmentation was becoming increasingly difficult because Army active and reserve medical forces were supporting protracted operations in both OIF and OEF. On behalf of LRMC, US Army Europe submitted a request for forces, asking for joint augmentation to staff the DWMMC and other areas within LRMC. In November 2006, the US Navy was tasked with fulfilling the request and responded with a reserve component Navy fleet hospital from Great Lakes, Illinois, with more than 300 assigned personnel. Since then, the Navy component at LRMC evolved into a Navy Expeditionary Medical Unit (NEMU). In 2007, other units evolved to support the wounded warriors:

- the *Medical Transient Detachment*: responsible for accountability of all outpatients and billeting (see Chapter 4, Medical Transient Detachment); and
- the *Chaplain's Closet*: provided clothing and personal items for soldiers, such as food, DVDs, CDs, and books (later realigned under the responsibility of LRMC chaplains; see the "Chaplain's Closet" vignette in Chapter 9, Chaplain Services).

IMPLEMENTATION METHODS

Organization and Responsibilities of the Deployed Warrior Medical Management Center

The DWMMC was composed of a command and control section and four departments (Operations, Nursing, Logistics, and Clinic). The LRMC deputy commander for clinical services had operational control of the DWMMC, while administrative control of Navy personnel within DWMMC remained with the NEMU. In command and control roles, DWMMC had a total of five personnel: (1) the officer in charge, (2) the assistant officer in charge, (3) the staff noncommissioned officer in charge, (4) a civilian administrative assistant, and (5) a civilian data analyst. The officer in charge and the assistant officer in charge positions were filled by both Navy Medical Corps and Navy Medical Service Corps officers. Key command and control tasks included the following:

- manpower management,
- data analysis,
- process improvement,

- interagency communication,
- briefings and tours (as requested),
- personnel evaluations and awards, and
- subordinate and peer career development.

Organization of the Deployed Warrior Medical Management Center

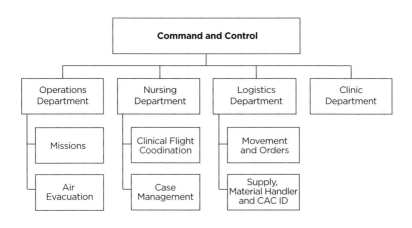

CAC ID: Common Access Card Identification

Courtesy of the Deployed Warrior Medical Management Center, Landstuhl Regional Medical Center.

OPERATIONS DEPARTMENT

This department consisted of 21 personnel, including a senior enlisted department head, and was divided into two branches: (1) Missions and (2) Air Evacuation. The Missions branch was the only office within DWMMC opened 24 hours a day, 7 days a week. It consisted of twelve military enlisted and one civilian personnel. This branch was responsible for the following:

- maintaining visibility and informing LRMC of inbound patients,
- registering and updating patients in medical information systems,
- coordinating patient reception,
- ensuring accountability, and
- providing orientation at reception.

The Air Evacuation branch was responsible for overseeing medical regulation of US military OCO patients designated for transfer to continued care (TCC) to CONUS in accordance with DoD and service-specific policies. The Air Evacuation branch had six military enlisted and one civilian personnel.

NURSING DEPARTMENT

This department consisted of nine military registered nurses (RNs), one of whom also served as department head, and five civilian RNs. This department also had two branches: (1) Clinical Flight Coordination (CFC) and (2) Case Management (CM). All of the military RNs worked in the CFC branch. They triaged all inbound OCO inpatients in consultation with on-call physicians prior to patients' arrival at LRMC, coordinated bed management of inpatients with LRMC Nursing Services, and entered consults for outpatients. CFC nurses also facilitated onward TCC movement through clinical review of medical information systems and outpatient interviews, entering necessary clinical information into PMRs.

The CM branch maintained continuity of information in medical information systems for both outpatients and inpatients and ensured that each US Army and Air Force wounded warrior outpatient completed his or her physician-developed treatment plan. CM referred patients for further evaluation if any concerns were identified during encounters. The Liaison Noncommissioned Officer (LNO) detachment at LRMC provided similar care coordination services for all Navy and Marine Corps patients. PAD provided CM for US government civilians, contractors, and coalition OCO patients.

LOGISTICS DEPARTMENT

This department consisted of 15 personnel, including a senior enlisted department head, and was divided into two sections: (1) Movement and Orders (M&O) and (2) Supply, Material Handler, and CAC ID. Staffed with seven enlisted military personnel, M&O prepared travel orders and coordinated commercial air transportation for Army wounded warriors designated for TCC or return to duty. It also coordinated ground transportation to the appropriate air terminal, military or commercial, for all departing patients or attendants. Its Navy, Marine Corps, and Air Force LNOs provided travel orders and commercial air coordination services for their respective patients (PAD provided similar services to US government civilians, contractors, and coalition OCO patients).

The Supply, Material Handler, and CAC ID section received, stored, issued, and disposed of inpatient and outpatient baggage and equipment. Additionally, this section operated a DEERS (Defense Enrollment and Eligibility Reporting System)/RAPIDS (Real-Time Automated Personnel Identification System) system to reissue lost or damaged military ID cards to patients supporting OCO and unlocked ID cards and verified certificates for LRMC staff. This section had two military enlisted personnel, four civilians, and one contractor.

CLINIC DEPARTMENT

This department served the primary care needs of all wounded warrior outpatients, performed medication reconciliation, ensured that traumatic brain injury screening was recorded, if appropriate, and provided sick call for NEMU personnel. The clinic consisted of four personnel, including one military physician (who also served as department head), one military physician assistant, one civilian physician assistant, and one military enlisted medic.

DEPLOYED WARRIOR MEDICAL MANAGEMENT CENTER CAPACITY

At the height of the war, 60 DWMMC triservice and civilian staff sustained a throughput (reception plus onward movement) of approximately 1,700 patients per month through the consolidation of critical clinical and administrative functions, as described below. This ensured efficient and effective coordination of the needs of the wounded warriors.

Prearrival

Patients from downrange arrived on evacuation flights at Ramstein Air Base. The Missions branch was responsible for monitoring TRAC2ES every hour to identify all evacuation flights destined for LRMC within the next 24 hours. Depending on the number of casualties, DWMMC usually received one to two flights per day, except for during the height of the war when there may have been three or four. Once an inbound flight became visible, the following sequence of events occurred:

- The Missions branch began registering patients on the flight in the Composite Health Care System and notified CFC.
- CFC nurses reviewed the PMRs and TMDS to begin prearrival triage. CFC nurses consulted either the internal medicine or general surgery on-call physician, depending on the patient's diagnosis.
- The on-call internal medicine or general surgery physician determined to which specialty service each inpatient would be admitted.
- CFC nurses then notified the designated specialty service and the wards to ensure that they were prepared to receive the patient.
- The DWMMC Clinic department head reviewed the PMRs to ensure that each outpatient had enough medication to last until his or her first appointment with a specialty provider.
- Once admitting service designation and ward assignment of inpatients were completed, CFC nurses notified the Missions branch, which finalized the inbound patient manifest.

- The Missions branch electronically posted the inbound patient manifest on both the DWMMC network drive and on the STARTC (Soldier Transfer and Regulating Tracking Center) Army Knowledge Online

Patient Flow Through the Deployed Warrior Medical Management Center

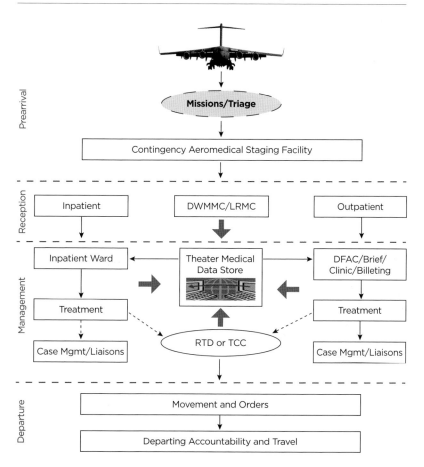

DFAC: Dining Facilities Administration Center
DWMMC: Deployed Warrior Medical Management Center
LRMC: Landstuhl Regional Medical Center
Mgmt: Management
RTD: return to duty
TCC: transfer to continued care

Courtesy of the Deployed Warrior Medical Management Center, Landstuhl Regional Medical Center.

page. The Missions branch then notified the appropriate personnel teams who were responsible for meeting the ambulance buses arriving from the Contingency Aeromedical Staging Facility at Ramstein Air Base to offload inpatients.

Reception

The condition and number of patients on each inbound flight determined the need for the number of medical ambulance buses. A Missions branch representative, a CFC nurse, and LRMC teams met each evacuation flight on arrival, and the patients were transported by ambulance bus to LRMC. The job of the Missions branch was to ensure accountability, whereas the CFC nurse received clinical updates from Contingency Aeromedical Staging Facility personnel. If significant changes in a patient's status had occurred, the CFC nurse retriaged the patient to make a final decision on the appropriate medical plan. Each inpatient was offloaded by the team and taken by the appropriate personnel to his or her respective wards. Outpatients met with their respective LNOs and were assigned to the Medical Transient Detachment.

Management

The primary care needs of US military OCO outpatients and their escorts were met by the DWMMC clinic, which provided primary care services, medication refills, and sick call, also ensuring that traumatic brain injury screening was complete.[2] Each outpatient was required to report to CM following every specialty appointment. The DWMMC CM was then responsible for the following:

- ensuring that consults were completed;
- generating a weekly report intended to maintain visibility of patient flow in accordance with theater evacuation policy;
- entering outpatient encounters in the Armed Forces Health Longitudinal Technology Application (AHLTA);
- collaborating with the physicians, command liaisons, the service member's command, and the DWMMC clinic for coordinating every aspect of wounded warrior care; and
- entering inpatient information from Essentris (the inpatient electronic medical record system) into TMDS, which provided visibility to deployed unit leadership and augmented information continuity (access to this medical information was helpful to the providers who cared for these soldiers after LRMC, when they are treated in US hospitals or by the Veterans Administration).

Departure

There were two possible dispositions for each OCO patient who was received at LRMC: (1) TCC or (2) return to duty. The average length of stay at LRMC was 3 to 5 days for inpatients and 10 days for outpatients.[2] For TCC patients, the following steps were performed:

- The attending specialist at Landstuhl initiated Form AF IMT 3899 PMR and submitted it to the DWMMC Air Evacuation branch.
- The Air Evacuation branch created a PMR in TRAC2ES, completed the administrative sections, and forwarded it to the CFC nurses.
- CFC nurses then accessed inpatient and outpatient electronic medical records to enter the necessary clinical information onto the PMR.
- CFC nurses also conducted interviews with outpatients designated for TCC. The CFC nurses compiled patient medical data, including transcribing data from Essentris and AHLTA, the Composite Health Care System, TMDS, and previous PMRs. The CFC nurses also coordinated with the validating flight surgeon at the Theater Patient Movement Requirements Center, Europe, regarding onward movement via commercial or military air travel.
- M&O issued temporary change of station orders for Army patients who were either TCC or return to duty, and then created and distributed bus manifests and TCC reports.
- M&O also coordinated with the DoD-contracted travel company for commercial air travel of wounded warriors.

Deployed Warrior Medical Management Center Equipment

DWMMC required no specialized equipment beyond standard office spaces and workstations. The following is a list of recommended information systems that required access and proficiency in use:

- TRAC2ES,
- TMDS,
- AHLTA,
- Composite Health Care System,
- Essentris,
- Medical Protection System,
- Single Mobility System,
- DEERS,
- Defense Medical Logistics Standard Support,
- Army Knowledge Online, and
- Automated Orders and Resource System.

Deployed Warrior Medical Management Center Reports

The DWMMC prepared and distributed a number of regular and ad hoc reports. Recurring LRMC internal reports included a daily morning report; weekly, monthly, quarterly, and fiscal year LRMC patient movement summaries; and inbound patient manifests (as required). Recurring external reports included outbound patient manifests, bus manifests, TCC reports, and Office of The Army Surgeon General reports. The DWMMC officer in charge and Clinic department head met weekly to review all outpatients who were at LRMC for 10 days or more to ensure compliance with theater evacuation policy.

LESSONS LEARNED

Since 2004, LRMC has received and treated more than 70,000 patients evacuated from OCO.[3] LRMC achieved an approximate 20% return-to-duty rate, which is significantly higher than in any previous conflicts.[3] More than 14,000 of these patients were treated as a result of battle injuries, and 85% of these patients spent less than 96 hours at LRMC prior to TCC to CONUS.[3] Both the PAD and the DWMMC significantly contributed to the efficient reception and movement of patients. This led to reduced loss of personnel to deployed units, cost avoidance from reduction of necessary TCC to CONUS, and improved outcomes through case managed and coordinated care. These benefits were seen at the unit level, the service component level, and the DoD level.

Successes and Challenges for the Patient Administration Division

- An early lack of compliance oversight and coding training for providers and coders was resolved through the development of the Training, Auditing, and Compliance branch, which provided coding training for providers and certification for new coders.
- Locating housing for foreign military and US civilian employees and contractors requiring outpatient treatment, who did not qualify for lodging and support at the hospital, was often problematic. PAD's solution was to acquire rooms in local billeting on an ongoing basis.
- Foreign patients who required a visa to enter Germany encountered immigration problems, which were resolved by developing a mechanism through the German Interior Ministry for pre-approval delivery of passports to the German federal police.
- Communication with foreign patients and their home governments was challenging. This situation was improved by establishing and supporting a foreign medical liaison program whereby liaisons were translators and conduits for communication with their home nations and military organizations.

Deployed Warrior Medical Management Center Successes

- The DWMMC has a proven outcome of decreasing the length of stay for wounded warriors from deployed units, limiting time spent at LRMC to 14 days or less for outpatients. The DWMMC directly contributed to the approximate 20% return-to-duty rate for those evacuated from theater.[3]
- A DWMMC could be set up at any medium-to-large medical treatment facility, provided extra required staff and equipment are available to deal with a recurring influx of patients during a conflict. It is also conflict-adaptable and can be altered, depending on the needs of the patients being evacuated from theater. The records of this process and skill sets must be maintained to ensure efficiency of medical care and evacuation channels in any future conflicts.
- DWMCC processes were replicated and perfected to the point that most were second nature within the hospital. The number of inbound and outbound OCO patients were included as part of the morning command report. This innovative idea was generated specifically for LRMC and to date has not been replicated at any other post. It has proved successful for LRMC and is clearly a best practice for contingency missions.
- A summary of DWMCC successes include the following:
  — worldwide availability of patient movement information;
  — patient reception and accountability;
  — coordinated cooperative reception with multiple teams, including LNOs, chaplains, DWMMC personnel (Missions and CFC branches), and LRMC personnel teams;
  — seamless patient handoff from LRMC to the Contingency Aeromedical Staging Facility;
  — CM services that ensured continuity of care; and
  — continuous information flow and in-transit visibility for both the receiving medical treatment facilities and the deployed unit leadership.

Deployed Warrior Medical Management Center Challenges

- *Lack of training.* There was no DWMMC-specific predeployment training for assigned Navy, Army, or Air Force personnel. Additionally, DoD patient movement and service-specific medical regulating policies and related information systems were generally not well known, except in particular specialties or communities. As a result, the staff experienced a steep learning curve. The curve may be reduced by implementing sufficient turnover periods between rotations.

- *Regulations and policy updates.* Because medical regulation policy updates were not always contiguous, DWMMC and clinical staff often questioned whether pre-existing policies were still to be used even when they were expired. Regulations and changes in such policies also needed to be explained to patients and families to help manage expectations.

- *Frequency of staff turnover.* Staff turnover within both the DWMMC and LRMC generated a particular challenge. The officer-in-charge position rotated more frequently than the rest of the DWMMC staff (usually every 6 or 9 months vs 12 months), and there were no civilians in leadership positions who could provide significant continuity across rotations. Because of the unpredictability of the number of casualties, DWMMC civilian positions were term, not permanent. Hiring was dependent on the limited local civilian talent pool. Furthermore, when LRMC staff experienced turnover, DWMMC had to engage in repeated education and expectation management for new providers and support staff who were unfamiliar with medical regulation policies, CENTCOM guidance, and the DWMMC scope of responsibility and authority. Each time new DWMMC personnel reported, there was friction for a period of time until rapport with the LRMC staff, the Contingency Aeromedical Staging Facility, the Theater Patient Movement Requirements Center–Europe, and STARTC were developed.

- *Ongoing change.* The DWMMC constantly evolved with ongoing improve-ment initiatives, changing service and combatant command policies, and changes in requests for feedback support. Although change was good, it needed to be carefully managed to reduce potential friction.

- *Funding multiple operations.* Funding of temporary change-of-station orders for soldiers from other than OEF and OIF was problematic. Specifically, DWMMC only had authorization to use budgetary funding associated with the aforementioned operations. However, there were other OCOs supported by LRMC and DWMMC, such as Operation Joint Guardian and Operation Joint Forge in EUCOM, and Combined Joint Task Force–Horn of Africa in AFRICOM.

- *Medical support of multiple operations.* LRMC supported OCO in three geographic combatant commander's AORs, but also supported non–OCO-eligible beneficiaries from those same AORs. DWMMC was created entirely for the support of OCO patients and was funded accordingly. LRMC PAD supported all non-OCO patients arriving at LRMC for care. It was not always clear whether an inbound flight or a patient was OCO or not. For example, LRMC received US military patients from embassies in CENTCOM or AFRICOM who at first glance were recognized as OCO, but in reality were not personnel on OCO deployment orders. DWMMC's practice was to treat all inbound flights and patients as OCO until definitively determined otherwise. When patients were determined to be other than OCO, DWMMC contacted the appropriate responsible party.

ACKNOWLEDGMENTS

Thanks to Commander Paul Pruden, DWMMC Assistant Officer in Charge; Lieutenant Darren Kasai, DWMMC Senior Noncommissioned Officer in Charge; HMCS (SW) Rachel Watson, DWMMC SNCOIC; LTC Weyman Cannington, Chief, Patient Administration Division; and Jeffrey Frazier, Deputy Chief, Patient Administration Division.

REFERENCES

1. Landstuhl Regional Medical Center Patient Administration Division. *How to be a Strategic Level IV MEDCEN Across the Spectrum of Conflict*. Landstuhl, Germany: LRMC; undated.
2. Landstuhl Regional Medical Center Public Affairs Office. *Fact Sheet: Deployed Warrior Medical Management Center*. Landstuhl, Germany: LRMC; October 2013.
3. Landstuhl Regional Medical Center Public Affairs Office. Medical Transient Detachment Sidebar [news release no. 11]. Landstuhl, Germany: LRMC; April 22, 2008.

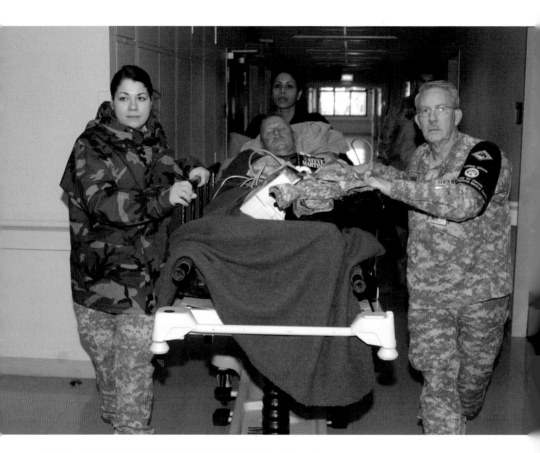

Liaison officer (*right*) escorts patient to the intensive care unit.

CHAPTER THREE

Liaisons

"The best way to find yourself is to lose yourself in the service of others."

— MAHATMA GANDHI

At any given moment at any location on the campus of Landstuhl Regional Medical Center (LRMC), a wounded warrior may hear these words: "if you have any questions or problems, ask your unit LNO (liaison officer)." An Army military article best described this position as follows: "Soldiers have their battle buddies. Airmen have their wingmen. Sailors have their shipmates. At LRMC, wounded warriors have their unit LNOs." [1]

The term "liaison" at its essence, refers to communication and cooperation maintained between elements of military forces or other agencies to ensure mutual understanding and unity of purpose and action. The liaison officer at Landstuhl Regional Medical Center (LRMC) is the official "go-between" serving as a critical point of contact for the patient, the patient's downrange unit and home station, and the patient's family. More than 30 Liaison Noncommissioned Officers (LNOs) from each service work with individual wounded warriors and play a critical role in their care. Liaisons escort wounded warriors to appointments, answer questions, and address a variety of their needs. Liaisons serve as a single point of contact and interface between LRMC and the medical department representatives of operational forces. This position is not a 0730 to 1630 job, but a way of life 24 hours a day, 7 days a week, 365 days a year.

The mission of Army liaisons is as follows: *To ensure that all wounded warriors receive the best care available and that they are returned to their home of record or placed in the closest medical treatment facility that has the capability to treat their injuries.* [2]

IMPLEMENTATION METHODS

What does it mean to be available 24 hours a day, 7 days a week? The role of the liaison begins before the patient arrives at LRMC and does not end until after the patient leaves. LNOs are the "master coordinators"; nothing is out of their job description. A liaison's duties can range from patient advocate and patient administrator, to counselor, finance clerk, driver, tour guide, first sergeant, and friend. The LNO is the one *consistent* person who wounded warriors can rely on. Reassurance is essential; while some soldiers are independent, others need hand-holding every step of the way. One LNO made the following remark:

> *In one hour, I may be picking up baggage, taking soldiers to appointments, picking up families at the airport, communicating with downrange units, tracking down a missing meal card, and running to Subway to get a sandwich for an inpatient soldier.*

The LNO offices are located in the multilevel trailer units that were built to accommodate the multiple administrative roles needed during the wars. LNOs, however, are rarely in those offices. They are constantly talking, moving, and multitasking. While the job entails a great deal of unpredictability, what every LNO does know for sure is that no moment can ever be wasted.

Liaison Force Structure

LNOs are assigned to LRMC by their respective units. During the height of the war, there were more than 40 LNOs responding to the three to five flights coming in per day from Iraq and Afghanistan. Some countries had their own LNO for coalition patients. If this was not the case, PAD (Patient Administration Division) assigned an LNO for those patients as well. Although the numbers of LNO personnel needed to staff the various branches has fluctuated over the years in response to war needs and demands (from 7 to 40), the liaison force structure for all military branches, *on average*, has included the following:

- *Army Liaison Force Structure.* Army liaisons have 26 members paired up to cover their respective post assignments. Army LNOs are deployed to LRMC from 6 months to 1 year. Army liaisons include two National Guard LNOs and four Reserve LNOs; 18 of them are active duty, including a senior Army LNO, for a total of 24 LNOs.
- *Air Force Liaison Force Structure.* The Air Force has two liaisons deployed to LRMC. Both are enlisted positions filled by either reservists or active duty service members. These service members are deployed to LRMC for 150 to 179 days. One of the Air Force liaisons also serves as the noncommissioned officer in charge (NCOIC) of the 86th Medical Squadron's Deployer Flight.
- *Navy Liaison Force Structure.* The Navy Liaison Office is a detachment from other naval hospitals across Europe who have been reassigned to

represent the Navy as LNO officers at LRMC. All four LNO sailors are on 3-year permanent change-of-station orders. The four Navy LNO personnel are: (1) chief hospital corpsman (FMF [Fleet Marine Forces]), officer in charge, Navy Liaison Detachment; (2) hospital corpsman first class (FMF), lead petty officer; (3) hospital corpsman second class (FMF), Navy liaison; and (4) hospital corpsman second class, Navy liaison. All Navy liaisons are active duty. All sailors in the Navy Liaison Office are trained in the same manner from top to bottom. This ensures that the care provided to wounded sailors and Marines is the same across the board.

- *Marine Liaison Force Structure.* The Landstuhl Marines are a detachment of Wounded Warrior Battalion–East, based out of Camp Lejeune, North Carolina. The nine Marine liaisons, all reservists, are deployed on 2-year, permanent change-of-station orders. The religious ministry team attached to the Marine liaison team has one Navy chaplain and one chaplain's assistant (an E-5; religious program specialist second class).

Liaison Duties

Duties of the liaison include the following:

- tracking inbound patients,
- meeting new patients,
- monitoring patients by keeping daily track of their whereabouts and medical progress,
- assisting patients,
- assisting families of patients,
- assisting discharged patients,
- assisting other liaisons and agencies, and
- providing communication.

TRACKING INBOUND PATIENTS

Continual monitoring of all inbound and outbound aeromedical evacuation traffic occurs through the TRANSCOM Regulating and Command & Control Evacuation System (TRAC2ES). Liaisons meet every flight to receive the patients. Planning and preparing for patient arrivals and departures are challenges that demand extensive flexibility for the LNO because of the dynamic nature of flight schedules and changing patient conditions. The liaison must sort out who is here for what reason, and correctly identify arriving patients by service branch, as well as any attendants who are accompanying them. The LNO is responsible for the whereabouts of all medical patients and non-medical escorts on the flight manifest in TRAC2ES. Liaisons must also make special arrangements and notifications for distinguished visitors (DVs) who come to LRMC to meet with the patients and tour the facility. Every DV has an LNO assigned to them, paired by military branch of service.

The Deployed Warrior Medical Management Center (DWMMC) mission team provides a finalized manifest via e-mail and contacts liaisons approximately 2 hours in advance of flight arrival. Flights are scheduled from several downrange bases and do not arrive on a particular schedule. Liaisons meet flights at various times throughout the day and night, depending on aeromedical evacuation patient requirements, aircraft availability, and weather conditions.

The liaison enters information on every identified inbound patient into the database and prepares an arrival information package. This requires researching the aeromedical evacuation mission's information in TRAC2ES and researching the TRAC2ES patient medical record. The purpose of this initial data collection is to understand the patient's condition and needs, to prepare for any special requirements, to establish downrange and home station communication, and to amend the daily status of patient reports for several chains of command throughout the Department of Defense.

LRMC also receives "ghost" patients on an unpredictable basis. Ghost patients refer to those soldiers, contractors, etc, stationed in other areas of the world (ie, other parts of Europe, Africa, and Egypt) who are in need of medical care or evaluation, and their location of deployment lacks this capability. They are therefore sent to LRMC for care, but they are not patients normally tracked by local patient administration or who are within the aeromedical evacuation system. Ghost patients arrive unexpectedly and require "work on the fly" to address their needs because they are not tracked in TRAC2ES. They typically arrive via normal military air rotations from downrange or, in some cases, via commercial air. LNOs must then ensure that transportation is provided to and from the Ramstein Passenger Terminal and Frankfurt Airport.

MEETING NEW PATIENTS

Regardless of time of day or any weather condition, each liaison is present to meet the AMBUS (ambulance bus) on arrival in front of the hospital. The liaison meets individually with each patient (and escort, if required), provides a personal briefing, collects all required information, identifies any initial needs, and establishes rapport. This initial meeting often sets patients at ease and provides a sense of comfort knowing that another soldier, airman, sailor, or Marine is there for them at all times.

Initial needs vary by patient, but may include some of the following:
- provision of a CAC (Common Access Card),
- reception,
- post exchange vouchers,

- finance support,
- uniforms and physical training gear,
- baggage,
- clothing,
- toiletries and other items,
- lodging,
- tours,
- contacting next of kin,
- escorting to an initial appointment, and
- addressing emergent care requirements.

Once initial needs are addressed, the liaison advises the patient to stay in contact with his or her family, deployed unit leadership, and home station leadership. It is vitally important that the patient do so because liaisons are heavily restricted by HIPAA (Health Insurance Portability and Accountability Act) privacy laws.

In the event that a ghost patient arrives, the liaison must escort this person through the entire DWMMC process, including all in-processing. The liaison must also escort the patient to the Medical Transient Detachment (MTD) or, in the case of a DV, to the Fisher House or Ramstein Inn to establish billeting. The liaison must also coordinate initial appointments for these patients. When LRMC receives a DV, the liaison must make lodging and transportation arrangements, and contact appropriate personnel (including LRMC Public Affairs) to ensure that hospital leadership is aware and available, as necessary. The liaison also escorts the patient to and from appointments and addresses all other needs.

MONITORING PATIENTS

Patients are tracked daily by liaisons. The liaisons are responsible for knowing where each patient is housed, monitoring the attendance of all scheduled visits, and following their progression of care. To track patient care and keep it moving forward, liaisons are responsible for the following:

- contacting the patient directly;
- accessing the Theater Medical Data Store (TMDS) to view appointments (when updated), working with DWMMC Case Management to access the Armed Forces Health Longitudinal Technology Application (AHLTA) to determine the medical status of the patient; and
- contacting a particular inpatient ward for updates (neither liaisons nor Case Management have access to Essentris, the inpatient electronic medical record system).

Liaisons visit every inpatient daily. Patients are often housed in rooms alone with limited access to the outside world. Liaisons help bridge this gap by checking on the patient's care and providing a listening ear. This is especially valuable for those patients undergoing specialty care not available at LRMC, but at other German civilian hospitals (ie, Saarland University Medical Center, Homberg, or University Hospital Regensburg) because a liaison is often the only American face they will see during their stay.

Liaisons also keep track of the whereabouts of all *nonmedical* patient attendants (escorts) and provide nearly the same services for them as well. They serve in an oversight role to make sure that patients and escorts meet their obligations, such as attending all required appointments (including physically escorting patients to their appointments, as needed) and complying with all LRMC and MTD rules. Liaisons ensure patient and escort accountability, and coordinate administrative action with downrange leadership and home station leadership. This often requires liaisons to physically track down patients to get them to wherever they are required to be at any given point in time.

ASSISTING PATIENTS

The liaison assists patients for specific reasons, such as the following:

- Escorting them to and from scheduled appointments, which is especially critical for patients undergoing sedation. The liaisons must remain with patients for the extent of the appointment. This responsibility also includes appointments at Ramstein Air Base (typically dental) and at civilian hospitals in the area for specialty care not available at LRMC.
- Escorting patients requiring additional medical attention (those with limited movement or who are wheelchair bound, etc).
- Obtaining prescribed medications.
- Acquiring necessities, such as toiletries, clothing, snacks, books, etc, from the Chaplain's Closet (see Chapter 9, Chaplain Services), the hospital shopette, or Ramstein Base Exchange.
- Locating patients' baggage from storage or following up on missing baggage with local baggage handlers, local and downrange contingency aeromedical staging facilities, and airlines.
- Transporting patients to and from Ramstein Air Base, local community services, and Frankfurt Airport.
- Helping patients replace a CAC.
- Helping patients address Government Travel Card loss.
- Working with Personnel Support for Contingency Operations (PERSCO) and downrange units to obtain patients' military orders.

This is particularly difficult when dealing with classified orders, because the liaison must coordinate Secret Internet Protocol Router Network (SIPRNET) communication and printing with Ramstein Medical Readiness.

ASSISTING FAMILIES OF PATIENTS

Sometimes a patient's medical condition necessitates bringing his or her family to visit for a given amount of time. The liaison coordinates emergency family medical travel via points of contact in Washington, DC. The liaison is then assigned to those family members for the entire duration they are at LRMC and provides one-on-one support. They ensure that family members have transportation, lodging, food, compassionate care, and assistance from appropriate caregivers. The liaison is responsible for the following:

- making billeting arrangements (a room is reserved at the Fisher House prior to their arrival for families visiting a seriously injured recovering warrior) so that families are close to their loved ones and are provided with a comfortable environment where they can share a common bond with others experiencing similar challenges;
- transporting the family to and from Frankfurt Airport;
- escorting the family to the patient;
- transporting the family to other services (for food, personal needs, etc.);
- helping with arrangements in the event of the patient's death;
- ensuring that the recovering warriors have contacted family members by phone, e-mail, or both; and
- arranging both pastoral care and holistic recovery services.

The patient and his or her family are the highest priority for the liaison, who establishes a unique rapport with both. The liaison is the face of the US military and is there to help families cope with a variety of circumstances.

ASSISTING DISCHARGED PATIENTS

Once LRMC discharges a patient, the liaison helps that patient with out-processing. This includes the following:

- outprocessing at the MTD;
- acquiring additional baggage, if necessary;
- coordinating baggage storage and pickup;
- assisting with ground transportation;
- coordinating aeromedical evacuation with home station patient administration;

- coordinating individual body armor shipment (about a third of the outpatient soldiers arrive with their body armor)—this is an important part of the discharge processing because the armor is very expensive and both the soldier and LNO are responsible for keeping track of it;
- coordinating stateside aeromedical evacuation changes to meet patient or family needs; and
- providing the patient's downrange units with a patient release letter.

ASSISTING OTHER LIAISONS AND AGENCIES

Liaisons work daily with active duty, Army National Guard, and Army Reserve counterparts to improve patient understanding and navigation of medical and nonmedical processes associated with their care and benefits. When working with seriously injured patients and their families, especially those requiring in-depth support, liaisons often work across service lines to assist liaisons from other branches to meet mission requirements.

PROVIDING COMMUNICATION

"My phone never stops ringing." This is a statement that is likely to be made by every LNO at LRMC. The liaison serves as the central point of contact for all wounded warriors at LRMC in fielding calls and e-mails around the clock from downrange units, home stations, various commands, and patient families. Both units and families require real-time information and sometimes direct patient communication regarding the patient's care or status. Calls come in at all hours of the day and night for updates. The day starts in Afghanistan at 0700, which is 0500 in Germany. Families of wounded warriors often contact the Family Readiness Group, who in turn contacts the LNO to get information about their loved ones.

To help streamline this process, each liaison has a work cell phone, enabling contact 24 hours a day, 7 days a week, 365 days a year. Home Internet access is also needed to review both TRAC2ES and the daily status of patient reports. In the event that more thorough information is required to assist information requests, the liaison readily returns to the office, regardless of the time of day or night, to access available resources and immediately answer information requests.

Most importantly, liaisons meet with both inpatients and outpatients at LRMC and at civilian hospitals in the area to address their needs. Based on appointment and procedure scheduling, the liaison is often with patients any time during the day and night. As a courtesy, the liaison attempts to contact patient units to provide them with an LRMC point of contact. The assigned liaisons are responsible for contacting the units of every active duty, Guard, and reserve wounded warrior, including those in classified locations. Liaisons must rely on each patient to provide accurate point-of-contact information because it is all but impossible to know deployed points of contact for every unit. In the vast majority of patient encounters, however, the liaison is often researching point-of-contact information based on just a last name (often misspelled) for each patient, and utilizing Air Force and Army global directories to locate a telephone number or e-mail address.

Unfortunately, in some instances, the contact information is simply not available, and liaisons must stand by for the unit to reach out to them. Liaisons do attempt to reach out to the deployed unit base operator to attempt to find a phone number for the patient's unit. The liaisons then attempt to establish an appropriate point of contact (typically a commander, first sergeant, or supervisor). Liaisons do their best to keep everyone informed about patient status in a timely manner, via telephone and e-mail. The immediate needs of patients and families always take priority. Because of HIPPA communication limitations, liaisons also rely on the patients themselves, the vast majority of whom are ambulatory and cognizant, to communicate with their respective units and keep them apprised of their status.

Service-Specific Duties of Liaisons

- *Army Liaisons.* The Army line-of-duty letter for soldiers in the reserve and National Guard states that the injured soldier was seen and treated at LRMC. The soldier then has this letter to verify that he or she was seen for a specific ailment or injury. The line-of-duty letter ensures that any necessary follow-up care needed as a result of injury or ailment sustained during deployment is covered by the military if soldiers are re-deployed or visit their own primary care physician through TRICARE.
- *Air Force Liaisons.* Air Force liaisons maintain an ongoing relationship with the Ramstein recovery assistance coordinator, who is responsible for providing training, attending face-to-face meetings, and ensuring that communication flows back to patient home stations via recovery assistance channels. Liaisons also work with the Ramstein Airman and Family Readiness Center to help patients and families with other needs. Upon learning of the transfer of an injured airman, the Air Force liaison enters the new patient's name into the Air Force Wounded Warrior (AFW2) database and prepares an AFW2 arrival information package.
- *Navy Liaisons.* All wounded warriors who are returning on a military air MEDEVAC (medical evacuation) flight are required to have funded orders with a line of accounting. Outpatient travel for Navy and Coast Guard personnel are funded by the individual's command. Inpatient travel is chargeable to the US Navy Bureau of Medicine and Surgery. The Navy liaisons are provided a line of accounting at the beginning of

each fiscal year for the purpose of writing inpatient MEDEVAC orders for all Navy, Marine Corps, and Coast Guard personnel receiving care in Landstuhl. The Navy liaisons also act as medical case managers, providing daily medical updates to commands downrange via TMDS, e-mail, and telephone. Liaisons also work with LRMC providers to identify the receiving physicians in CONUS (continental United States), including the occasional civilian facility for Coast Guard patients, and to provide continuity of care.

- *Marine Liaisons.* Marine liaisons have a flight line escort specifically dedicated to arriving and departing Marine patients. The Marine LNO goes directly to Ramstein to receive the injured patients, rather than waiting for the AMBUS to arrive at LRMC. While the other service branch LNOs say good-bye to their patients at LRMC, the Marine LNO escorts them back to Ramstein to either return to their deployed units or transfer to CONUS. They also provide congressional notification forms to notify the injured Marine's congressperson and invitational travel order requests to the US Marine Corps Casualty Branch. In addition, they provide outpatient transfer orders for the patients. The US Marine Corps culture dictates that Marines care for each other as much as possible. The flight line liaison provides direct accountability at the earliest possible moment and provides a final handoff at the last possible moment.

ADDITIONAL TRACKING TOOLS

Liaisons frequently communicate with each other and rely on peer feedback to share ideas of "what works and what does not" in terms of the multiple demands and multitasking that is a part of their daily routine. LNOs also have access to a variety of different reports to track information on patients, including the following:

- patient air evacuation report,
- daily patient tracking report,
- host nation liaison report,
- daily departure report, and
- TRAC2ES.

LESSONS LEARNED

What is it that keeps pushing a person to keep going, to answer that 200th phone call, to coordinate just one more appointment, or to meet another AMBUS at 0500? Staff Sergeant Kevin Kirkpatrick, an LNO at LRMC, reflected a moment before answering that question:

On those really hard days when you are truly ready to collapse because you are just that dog tired; when you begin having mirage images of your own bed because you have put in so many hours and addressed so many needs, you do wonder what keeps you going. I thought I knew what "service" was. Then I came to Landstuhl, assigned as a liaison officer, and the word "service" took on a whole new dimension. This is real life and the real stuff of people's lives; nothing superficial. It is humbling and life-changing to hear so many stories from wounded warriors who never complain or question, "why me?" They will simply tell you they were serving their country and this is what happened. What keeps you going is the strength of the human spirit, the exchange of human connection, the humbling experience of seeing untold suffering and wondering why it is them and not you. It is a complete giving of self—service felt at a visceral level. And on those really hard days, that is what drives you to continue to do more.

It is impossible to overstate the liaison's importance to wounded warriors and their families. This role is a vital contribution to the success of the seamless flow at LRMC, and demands a wide range of professional and personal skills. The LNO is a person who needs to be highly organized and efficient, with navigational savvy, because he or she is required to access multiple systems and facilities throughout the Kaiserslautern Military Community and local area. Flexibility is essential because job responsibilities can vary from minute to minute, and schedules can dictate meeting patient and family needs at all hours of the day or night. The role of the LNO takes a great deal of maturity and personal strength to deal with unpredictable and sometimes difficult situations. Although all such skills are essential, empathy is perhaps the most important, because LNOs are people with the ability to continually offer that friendly smile even when they cannot recall the last time they closed their eyes.

Successes

- *Patient reception.* Depending on wind, weather, and international airspace permission, it can take anywhere from 7 to 10 hours to fly from Afghanistan to Germany. Ambulatory wounded warriors step off the AMBUS tired, hungry, and often sick or in pain. Seriously injured patients are on stretchers, some intubated and unable to communicate. The LNO is one of the first to greet the patients on arrival to LRMC and sets the tone for the duration of their stay until departure. This initial interaction provides a great deal of comfort and stability for wounded warriors. During the reception, the LNO explains the general process and what to expect while at LRMC. This time also allows the patients to ask any questions or share any concerns that they may have.

- *Efficient communication with parent and operational command.* In the past, LRMC was called the "land of the lost" because patients arrived there and were not heard from for days or weeks on end. Status updates were not provided, and downrange units were uncertain what was happening to their soldiers: if they were returning to their units or being transferred for continuous care. The liaison has changed all of that. Notification e-mails are now sent by the liaison to both the patient's downrange and home stations within 8 hours of the patient's arrival. Leadership is informed every step of the way as they are updated with the patient's medical and logistical status while at LRMC. If a decision is made to transfer a soldier to CONUS, both the unit and receiving hospital are frequently updated with medical status, flight itineraries, and when "wheels up" occurs. This reciprocal dialogue has been greatly appreciated by the patients and their units, and has alleviated much stress. Direct contact information is also given to the unit to be passed on to the patient's family. The patient is given access to call the home station or deployed units.

    The *Air Force LNO* notifies the Casualty Affairs Office of the patient's arrival and the names of family members requested to be at bedside, if applicable. Bringing family members to the patient's bedside in a timely manner is a team effort. There is a strong working relationship with the Casualty Affairs Office, which provides the orders enabling families to come to LRMC and ensures that expenses are covered.

Challenges

- *Patient attendants/escorts.* Certain circumstances require the need for an escort to accompany wounded warriors to LRMC. In the majority of situations, the escort is another soldier from the same downrange unit. The escort is usually told at the last minute that he or she is escorting a patient to LRMC and to come right back. The escorts and their units are often under the impression that they will be released immediately to return downrange once they have arrived with the wounded warrior at LRMC. It usually comes as a shock when they arrive at LRMC and are then told that they are not immediately returning, and are given other duties and responsibilities. There are situations in which patients need someone with them at all times because of a concern they could potentially harm themselves or other personnel. Even if

[handwritten margin note top: isn't it more important for deployed units to be fully strengthed?]

[handwritten margin note left: I feel that This is A Problem of Medical not understanding The Line]

the soldier is being treated as an outpatient, the escort needs to be with the soldier at all times. Other patients may need to be wheeled around to appointments or need help with getting or eating food, etc. Although the liaison is an extraordinary support to wounded warriors, the workload and the volume of patients do not realistically enable the liaison to address patient needs on a one-to-one basis. Downrange leadership needs to inform the escort of what will be expected of him or her *prior to arrival at LRMC.* Often, the liaison must deal with both the injured or sick soldier and a disgruntled escort.

- *External interference with the patient movement process.* In certain situations, unique arrangements are made by the patients themselves, which deviates from the LRMC standard operating procedures, thus making their accountability more difficult for the LNOs. For example, some patients do not adhere to standard procedures, such as taking bus transportation from the MTD to the passenger terminal; instead, they take it upon themselves to make their own travel arrangements. Other times, patients have their commander's permission to deviate from the process, such as flying out of Frankfurt Airport instead of Ramstein. This causes time away from the mission because the LNO is asked to make these special arrangements, accompany the patient to the specific airport, maintain accountability of that separate flight status, and track when that individual arrives at his or her destination.

- *Resiliency and compassion fatigue.* The liaison mission is maintained 24 hours a day, 7 days a week. At the height of the wars, or when attending to unusual circumstances or complications with wounded warriors, liaisons sometimes work 19 hours daily. There is very little to no "down time." This is both physically and emotionally stressful and exhausting. It is therefore imperative that LNOs work as a solid team, with seamless debriefings when duties are taken over to maintain mission continuity. Flexibility is key. A good working relationship leads to a good working schedule.

It is imperative for the LNOs to take the time to meet with the Combat and Operational Stress Reaction/Staff Resiliency Team. Although this is not a mandatory requirement, it is extremely beneficial given the constant stress and demands of the LNO and the LRMC staff in general. This team's mission is to promote resiliency and to identify and treat operational stress and compassion fatigue via prevention and intervention efforts. The important aspect for anyone seeking intervention is that the counseling is done on a one-to-one basis and remains confidential. This policy is particularly essential and has alleviated some of the reluctance of staff to meet and talk with the team for fear it would not remain private information. The Resiliency Team also arranges weekly game and pizza nights as a fun and relaxing event. This has been very popular.

- *High staff turnover/no current overlap time in place for training.* The LNOs are comprised of Army, Navy, Marine, and Air Force deployed personnel. All LNOs are deployed for 1 year, except the Air Force LNOs who are deployed for 6 months. It is crucial to ensure that overlap training is built into the deployment orders for the LNOs. With no overlap training, it could lead to degradation in the mission.

- *Lack of representation from all stateside units.* LNOs are deployed to LRMC from their stateside military bases to represent and serve those soldiers from their units who have been injured in the war and sent to LRMC for treatment. Some of the large US military units with many soldiers deployed to Iraq and Afghanistan have not, however, sent an LNO to serve at LRMC. This has been a challenge because every wounded warrior at LRMC is required to have an assigned LNO. The accountability and needs of these soldiers are then divided up among the LNOs from other units, which adds additional stress and time commitment. It is not as much of a problem for the smaller units without an LNO representative because the numbers of injured soldiers are proportionately less and therefore manageable. It is a much bigger challenge for the larger units sending hundreds of soldiers into theater, with a much higher percentage likely to arrive at LRMC for treatment of various sorts. The support of the LNO cannot be underestimated, and is particularly paramount when the injured solider comes off of the AMBUS and is greeted and reassured by an LNO from his or her home unit. It is like being greeted by an old friend, and immediately reduces stress and anxiety. Although soldiers from other units are given equal time and assistance, they feel disappointed that someone from their home unit is not there to support them. The importance of every US military unit sending representation is essential in terms of both workload and soldier morale.

ACKNOWLEDGMENTS

The authors would like to thank Lieutenant Colonel William Branch, Detachment Officer in Charge, US Marine Corps Wounded Warrior Battalion–East; Chief Master Sergeant Charles Frizzell, Senior Master Sergeant Gloria Portillo-Leanos, and Master Sergeant Philip Gilbert, US Air Force Liaisons; Lieutenant Colonel Brenda Corrunker, US Air Force; Master Sergeant Luis Sanchez, Senior Army Liaison; Staff Sergeant Kevin Kirkpatrick, US Army; and HMF (FMF) David Livesay, Officer in Charge, Navy/Marine Corps Fleet Liaison Detachment.

REFERENCES

1. Melancon D. Liaisons 'watch over' Landstuhl's wounded. May 25, 2007. US Army news website. http://www.army.mil/article/3343/Liaisons___039_watch_over__039__Landstuhl__039_s_wounded/. Accessed January 28, 2015.
2. Mission statement provided by Lieutenant Colonel Brenda Corrunker, US Air Force, Liaison, Landstuhl Regional Medical Center.

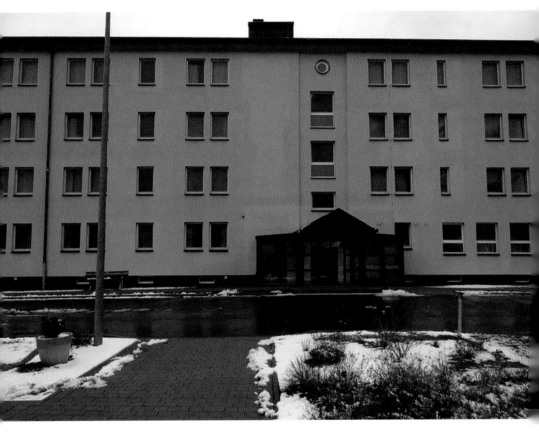

Medical Transient Detachment facility at Landstuhl Regional
Medical Center.

Photograph courtesy of Captain Marcus McGee, US Army.

CHAPTER FOUR

Medical Transient Detachment

"Servients Nostri Vulnerati" (Serving Our Wounded)

*I grew up in a family of 12 siblings, and all that I do is based on my
upbringing and family morals and traditions. If anyone needed assistance,
my family always made an effort to lend a helping hand because others
helped us when we were in need. That will always be instilled in me.
I treat everyone as I would like to be treated. I was hand-picked as
First Sergeant at the MTD [Medical Transient Detachment], and my
responsibility was to take care of those soldiers the best way I could.
I believed that all warriors deserved the best during their transition.
Every day, I personally asked every wounded warrior if they had an
anniversary or a birthday, and, if so, I recognized them in the formation.
This could have been embarrassing for some because we did sing
Happy Birthday. I also bought lunch or dinner out of my own pocket for
every wounded warrior who had a birthday while at the MTD. This was
my way of giving back to all who served in harm's way, for what they have
done, and for what they will continue to do.*

FIRST SERGEANT LARRY McGOWAN
LANDSTUHL REGIONAL MEDICAL CENTER, GERMANY
DECEMBER 2007–JUNE 2009

D riving along the campus at Landstuhl Regional Medical Center
(LRMC), one may not take particular notice of the two white stucco
buildings that blend in with the rest of the architecture. Yet these
buildings now represent an essential unit at Landstuhl, as well as one of the
most essential lessons learned during this war. Walking into the buildings is
like walking into a hotel: there is a warm and cozy sitting area with a television
adjacent to the reception desk, there is a smiling soldier extending a greeting, and
there is a glass jar filled with candy. It is not unusual to smell fresh coffee brewing

or freshly baked cookies coming out of the oven. One soldier commented that "this feels like the Taj Mahal compared to sleeping in a tent in the desert."

This renovated former Air Force hotel on the hospital premises is more like home, or at least pretty close to it. It is actually home to the Medical Transient Detachment (MTD), an organization responsible for overseeing the needs of those men and women who are in transient status while receiving outpatient care at LRMC. Although the actual physical structure was not renovated until 2007, the organization itself was established in 2003 with the responsibility of providing local mission command functions for soldiers, airmen, sailors, and Marines evacuated from Operation Iraqi Freedom (OIF), Operation Enduring Freedom (OEF), and Operation New Dawn. Although the MTD and Deployed Warrior Medical Management Center (DWMMC) are tightly linked and work in close coordination with each other, they are two separate organizations with separate leadership structures. Although the DWMMC tracks patient movement in the aeromedical evacuation system from downrange to Landstuhl and then coordinates the patient's medical and logistical needs, the DWMMC is not involved in overseeing each soldier on a daily basis.

While duty, honor, and responsibility encompass the backbone code of ethics of every infrastructure unit entrusted to care for the thousands of wounded warriors at LRMC, the MTD goes to a level of accountability even deeper than that. Each MTD cadre is responsible for tracking the whereabouts of *all of their patients, all day and every day*, regardless of rank or service affiliation. This daily proximity, constant interaction, and ongoing support lend themselves to a level of commitment and reciprocal personal impact that cannot be underestimated. Sergeant Major Larry McGowan states, "I wanted to provide the best care that I could based on my position and responsibility. I was able to listen to their stories of what they had gone through during their deployment and the reasons they were sent to Landstuhl. I participated in the group discussion of those soldiers with posttraumatic stress disorder (PTSD) and reassured them that things would get better. When soldiers didn't want to open up, I coached them as a senior leader, always reassuring them that what was said at the MTD would stay at the MTD."

The mission of the MTD is as follows: *To provide company-level mission command, administrative and logistical support, and quality of life needs to the evacuated wounded, ill, and injured service members, and all we are privileged to serve.*[1]

BACKGROUND

After creation of the DWMMC in 2002, it became apparent that a formal system of mission command was necessary for service members transferred to LRMC for outpatient care. In the summer of 2003, LRMC was inundated with sick and injured service members from OIF who needed the next role of medical treatment care. Not every soldier required inpatient care, and those who did not needed a place to stay. Initially, all outpatient wounded warriors were housed at Kleber Kaserne, the primary inprocessing/outprocessing center for the Kaiserslautern Military Community, and the location of the 21st Theater Sustainment Command (TSC). Kleber Kaserne had the capacity to house 300 patients in barracks. An entire building was designated to provide lodging for transient wounded warriors receiving outpatient care at LRMC. Although this facility provided the much-needed housing, the solution came at a logistical cost. Kleber Kaserne was 25 miles away from LRMC. This distance made both scheduling and attending appointments difficult for patients. It also limited the overall scope of command control. Staff members at LRMC were tasked with attending to the nightly charge of quarters on the billets housing these wounded warriors. This placed a heavy responsibility on staff lacking any true authority over these individuals.

Over time, LRMC was no longer able to maintain control and accountability of the continual large influx of evacuated patients from wars in Afghanistan and Iraq. Although the DWMMC was efficiently managing the process of bringing patients in and out of Landstuhl, it did not have the staff or command authority to deal with the increasingly problematic administrative and personnel issues. The DWMMC's authority was limited to patient care only. After several legal incidents, it became evident that a separate system for mission command specifically addressing the needs of these outpatients was necessary. Tasking soldiers to merely keep an eye on the patients did not work, and written policies were needed. Therefore, it was determined that some type of oversight was essential, and a formal system of mission command was required.

The MTD was then created in 2003 for this purpose. It was initially staffed with a commander, a first sergeant, five platoon sergeants, and three soldiers to perform administrative functions. During this time, the MTD was averaging a total of 180 to 200 outpatients, with daily in- and outprocessing of 20 to 40 personnel. In April 2004, during the First Battle of Fallujah in Iraq, Kleber Kaserne nearly reached its maximum occupancy of more than 280 soldiers, sailors, airmen, and Marines staying in the barracks while receiving care at LRMC. This was a daunting task for the MTD, which was staffed with only 10 personnel now overseeing nearly 300 patients.

Mission command of the MTD remained the responsibility of LRMC from 2003 to 2005. When it became increasingly problematic to provide available personnel for this level of patient support, the 21st TSC agreed to take on the role and provide mission command for patients evacuated to LRMC. Unfortunately, there was a lack of medical management and coordination between the 21st TSC and LRMC. Poor communication between personnel at LRMC and Kleber Kaserne resulted in patients missing appointments because they were either uninformed or simply did not show up. The MTD staffing at Kleber Kaserne was limited, and it was impossible for this small cadre to keep track of hundreds of patients effectively and make sure that they were following orders. Patients were assigned case managers, but the distance in location and poor communication also made it difficult for them to effectively and efficiently provide quality care. The culmination of these problems had further-reaching effects beyond the boundaries of LRMC and Kleber Kaserne. Downrange units were negatively impacted because there was no established timeline for returning these wounded warriors to duty. Outpatient stays were delayed at LRMC because of the lack of sufficient numbers of local mission command staffing and overall disorganization.

As time went on, it also became increasingly apparent that the lodging facilities were inadequate and contributed to the multiple problems. The 10-person, open-bay rooms at Kleber Kaserne were noisy and lacked privacy and comfort. The 30-minute bus commute to LRMC for appointments with doctors, therapists, liaisons, and case managers was inconvenient.[2] Morale and quality of life were adversely impacted by the limited amenities and suboptimal accommodations. It was clear that a new facility was needed to better serve patients and give them the dignity and care they deserved.

The current facility was renovated in 2007 on the grounds of LRMC, and the overall responsibility for the MTD unit was placed back under LRMC command. Outpatient soldiers were moved on post, now closer to their appointments. At this time, the Table of Distribution and Allowances—used for the Army Warrior Transition Units (WTUs)—was applied to the MTD to improve the cadre-to-patient ratios. It remains the current staffing structure used today.

IMPLEMENTATION OF MEDICAL TRANSIENT DETACHMENT
Leadership and Staffing
There is no other organization exactly like the MTD, although the Soldier Family Readiness Center at Walter Reed National Military Medical Center does replicate some functions handled at LRMC. WTUs replicate the MTD's local mission command function with a more long-term focus, whereas the MTD focuses on short-term support to all branches of the US military.

MTD leadership is comprised of a commander and a first sergeant. Their key tasks are to maintain the following:
- mission command of all assigned personnel;
- daily management of all MTD operations;
- continuous process improvement (a strategic approach to develop a culture of continuous improvement);

- joint coordination with DWMMC leadership, LRMC leadership, the Patient Administration Division, and various outpatient programs (eg, Traumatic Brain Injury, Intensive Outpatient Program for Post-traumatic Stress, Addiction Treatment Facility);
- personnel evaluations and awards; and
- subordinate and peer career development.

The MTD is aligned with the LRMC command structure, with direct reporting to the LRMC troop commander and the LRMC medical treatment facility commander. The remainder of the MTD staff includes the following:

- squad leader,
- platoon sergeants,
- civilian personnel, and
- liaison.

Medical Transient Detachment Structure

The MTD structure is much like the current WTU structure, but functions in a different manner. The MTD mission assists service members with either returning to duty or transferring to CONUS (continental United States) for continued care. Upon arrival at LRMC, the service member is assigned a liaison and an MTD squad leader, escorted to the outpatient facility for room assignment, and given an initial in-briefing regarding policies and procedures. The squad leader is responsible for coordinating efforts between the liaisons, DWMMC case managers, LRMC clinics, and MTD leadership to ensure that patients are well cared for and move through the system in an efficient and safe manner.

The platoon sergeants are, in turn, responsible for ensuring the accountability of all service members. This includes the patients evacuated to LRMC, the escorts who accompanied them, and the MTD cadre who provide support to the soldiers and carry out typical administrative duties. In addition, the MTD platoon sergeant and squad leaders are responsible for ensuring that all soldiers adhere to the MTD policies, such as the following:

- no drinking alcohol while assigned to the MTD;
- no overnight passes (exceptions made on case-by-case basis);
- day passes granted on a case-by-case basis;
- uniform adherence;
- computer adherence;
- daily morning and evening accountability;
- established curfew of 2300 hours (aligns with closing of USO [United Service Organization]);

- all service members restricted to MTD barracks between 2300 and 0600 hours;
- escorts must remain with appointed service member at all times;
- no outprocessing from the MTD without appropriate confirmation; and
- possession of contraband, drugs, ammunition, or illegal items is prohibited.[3]

The MTD has civilian personnel who issue vouchers and maintain the MTD's supply of clothing and personal care items. All US Army personnel receive a uniform issue if returning from downrange with missing items or unserviceable uniforms. They are often evacuated with very few belongings. The MTD is authorized to issue to all patients a one-time $250 Army and Air Force Exchange Service (AAFES) voucher that can be used to purchase personal care and clothing items from the local AAFES stores.[3]

Another civilian provides S-1 paperwork and administrative functions for both cadre and patients receiving care at LRMC. The first sergeant and commander provide overall mission command and also have the Uniform Code of Military Justice authority for all assigned and attached personnel.

The "gold standard" goal for anyone returning to CONUS is to provide necessary support and to complete an efficient and effective evacuation within 14 days. This is not an official policy, but rather a goal to strive for, especially during the height of the wars when bed space was at capacity. It is not always possible to attain because the length of hospital stay varies from patient to patient. Some patients have stayed as long as 8 weeks and were then ready to return to their units. Although every effort is made to return patients to active duty, some patients have to be returned to CONUS, where they have a support structure of family, friends, and the local command.

Medical Transient Detachment Capacity

The MTD has had anywhere from 27 to 34 Army and civilian personnel overseeing a facility that accommodates a maximum of 218 patients. It provides billeting and support services at any given time. When it was needed, additional overflow billeting was available at Landstuhl through coordination with the 21st TSC installation management office. Coordination with the DWMMC and patient liaisons enables the MTD to accommodate the DWMMC throughput, including processing patients from the time they arrive at Ramstein Air Base (Germany) to the time they leave LRMC and return to their unit or CONUS.

Medical Transient Detachment Equipment and Buildings

The MTD outpatient facility is a two-building, four-story structure transformed from a former Air Force hotel. The US Army Garrison Kaiserslautern Installation Management Command spent more than $2.9 million renovating the two buildings, which are located on the Landstuhl hospital grounds.[2] There are private rooms designated for senior personnel, and the remainder are two-person accommodations for a total capacity of 218 patients. Each room is generously equipped with one or two private beds, individual locking closets, a desk, microwave, mini-refrigerator, cable TV with a DVD player, telephone, and computer with free Wi-Fi Internet access and webcam capacity. There are also phones in the common area where patients can call anywhere in the world for free. Residents can prepare popcorn in their microwave and enjoy a cold soda from their mini-refrigerator while watching TV or e-mailing loved ones. They can also play video games in the community room, cook a meal in the fully furnished kitchen, or use the full-service laundry. It is not unusual for fresh-baked goods or donated food to appear in the refrigerator, compliments of many generous volunteers, all wanting to help soldiers feel at home.

ADDITIONAL RESOURCES AND SERVICES

- The MTD is responsible for overseeing transportation services between Landstuhl, Ramstein Air Base (location of base exchange/post exchange), and Kleber Kaserne (location of the Army clothing and sales store). There are scheduled bus trips every day to ensure that service members have opportunities to use clothing vouchers and have some downtime away from the medical center.
- The MTD coordinates efforts with the Chaplain Service, USO, Veterans of Foreign Wars, Soldiers' Angels, Red Cross, and other nonprofit organizations to organize scheduled bus trips to various cities and provide morale and welfare services dedicated to the service members staying in the MTD.
- The MTD also coordinates efforts with the LRMC command to provide mission command and lodging to the LRMC Addiction Treatment Facility, Evolution Posttraumatic Stress Disorder Treatment Program, Synapse Traumatic Brain Injury Program, and the Integrated Pain Management Center Program personnel.
- The MTD does not provide command and control or lodging services for foreign military personnel, civilians, or dependents.

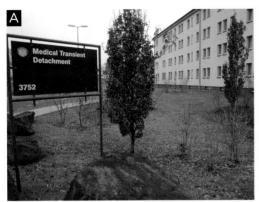
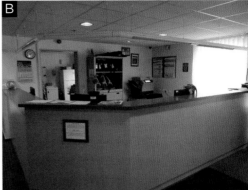
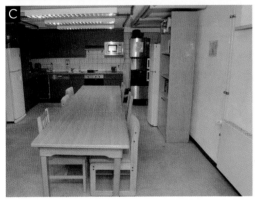
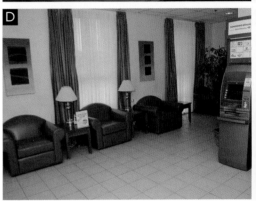

Views of the Medical Transient Detachment facility at Landstuhl Regional Medical Center: (A) building sign, (B) reception desk, (C) kitchen, and (D) lobby.

Photographs courtesy of Captain Marcus McGee, US Army.

LESSONS LEARNED

The MTD is an excellent example of a command structure that supports all branches of the services. The hospital has treated 61,155 patients evacuated from Iraq or Afghanistan, and 21% (12,691) of patients have returned to duty.[4] More than 12,000 patients have sustained battle injuries, and 85% of those patients are spending less than 96 hours at LRMC.[4] From 2007, when the building renovations were completed, to the end of 2013, more than 42,000 outpatients had gone through the MTD.[1] The fact that doctors, case managers, liaisons, Chaplain Services, and a wide circle of supporters are now just steps away has exponentially changed the dynamics of morale and overall quality of life for outpatient soldiers. Someone cares and is there to escort, listen, or lighten a burden at any corner they turn. This system of 24-hour accountability and proximal mission command dramatically increased the safety, security, stability,

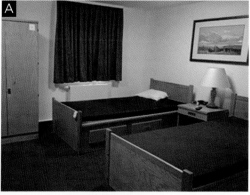
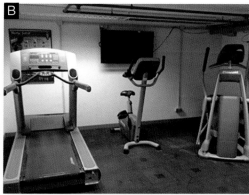
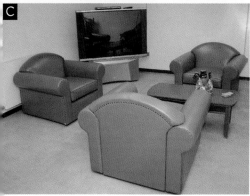
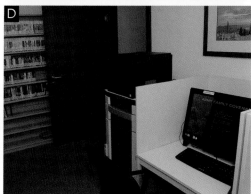

Life inside the Medical Transient Detachment offers some of the comforts of home: (A) bedroom, (B) exercise room, (C) common area and TV room, and (D) the Internet cafe.

Photographs courtesy of Captain Marcus McGee, US Army.

and success of patient care. The MTD has done an outstanding job, significantly contributing to the impressive mission at LRMC.

As the US military becomes smaller and military facilities are combined (eg, Walter Reed Army Medical Center with the National Naval Medical Center and the San Antonio Military Medical Center with the Wilford Hall Ambulatory Surgical Center), it is important that future leaders use the MTD command structure as an example of how to provide mission command support to patients from all service branches of the military.

Successes

- The MTD has a proven record of helping to decrease lost time from downrange units by limiting time spent at LRMC to 14 days or less and has directly contributed to the 21% return-to-duty rate for those evacuated from theater.[4]

- Outpatient lodging facilities on the Landstuhl grounds significantly cut costs (approximately $5–$6 million dollars/year from paying for accommodations for soldiers at the Ramstein Inn).[1]
- The MTD can be set up at any medium-to-large military medical treatment facility provided there are extra required staff and equipment to deal with the reoccurring influx of patients from a conflict.
- The MTD is a great example of how people come together to help those who are hurt and in need. There is a unified seamless flow of teamwork between all branches interacting and working together. Everyone benefits from the reciprocal understanding of each service branch and what they do.
- The MTD is conflict-adaptable and can be altered depending on the needs of the patients being evacuated from the theater of operations or in a garrison environment. This is perhaps its greatest strength.
- The MTD processes that serve its patient population have been institutionalized to the point that most processes are self-regulated within the hospital. It has been proven successful for LRMC, and is clearly a best practice for contingency missions and may be applicable to noncontingency missions in a garrison environment for future utilization.
- The mission command of the MTD ensures safety and security to soldiers receiving care, and is essential to maintaining good order and discipline. These benefits are seen at the unit, service component, and Department of Defense levels.

Challenges
- Justifying the existence of the MTD in a conflict-free military is a significant obstacle in maintaining the current operating structure and staffing levels.
- Although the MTD has focused primarily on the deployed soldiers, airmen, sailors, and Marines from Afghanistan, it may be necessary to use this same structure (and perhaps the same unit) to provide mission command and lodging for wounded military in the European area who currently travel to LRMC for outpatient specialty services unavailable in areas of Bavaria, Italy, and Belgium. If this is the future of the MTD, it is imperative that wounded warriors report for orders to the MTD (to maintain mission command) and are unaccompanied by family members when using the MTD services on a short-term basis (eg, specialty provider appointments, outpatient procedures, and MRIs [magnetic resonance imaging]).

Patients Transitioned Through the Medical Transient Detachment Since FY2007

YEAR	NUMBER OF PATIENTS
FY07	5,442
FY08	6,370
FY09	6,351
FY10	8,055
FY11	6,827
FY12	5,002
FY13	3,549
FY14	1,775
TOTAL	43,371

FY: fiscal year
Reproduced from: McGee M, Bond J. Medical Transient Detachment, Landstuhl Regional Medical Center, command brief. PowerPoint presentation; April 2014; LRMC, Germany.

- Some military hospitals may have barracks and buildings available, but are they logistically located? Do they provide optimal accommodations? It may be necessary to finance renovations of existing structures or build a new facility. This would pose a challenge, especially with fiscally tight budgets. Over the long term, however, it would save the government a lot of money with lodging costs.
- Keeping track of every wounded warrior for medical care, especially when they were not in transit, is a daunting task. Many still found ways to disobey orders and sneak away from the MTD and Landstuhl to go downtown and consume alcohol.
- Better training is needed to prepare those assigned to the MTD. Most of the soldiers come from an infantry unit and are used to being in the field. They are not familiar with medical knowledge or what it means for someone to be sick, scared, in pain, or in need of medical care. Many of these younger soldiers, both patient and personnel, have never been in a hospital. It can be an overwhelming process. The MTD would likely benefit from the 2-week WTU Cadre Training.

When Sergeant Larry McGowan was asked what he would remember the most about his time at Landstuhl working for the MTD, he responded with the following:

I will always remember October 31, 2008. I invited all those who supported the wounded warriors from LRMC and Ramstein to participate in the Costume Run. It was a moment that was frightening to the soldiers because the announcement over the public affairs system said for all of them to get out of their rooms. They were expecting me to bring drug dogs in the barracks. Instead, I had my staff, who were all dressed in costumes, turn out the lights and run through the barracks yelling "Trick or Treat" and passing out candy. We then invited those who were able to go for a run/walk. We actually pushed a wounded warrior in a wheelchair along the 2-mile route we ran. What I will remember is how important it was to find ways to make those wounded warriors laugh. It really was a place to heal at a home away from home.

ACKNOWLEDGMENTS

The author thanks Captain Daniel Yourk, First Sergeant Phillip Madrigal, Sergeant First Class Jeffrey Lawrence, and Captain Marcus McGee for their invaluable assistance with this chapter.

REFERENCES

1. McGee M, Bond J. Medical Transient Detachment, Landstuhl Regional Medical Center, command brief. PowerPoint presentation; April 2014; LRMC, Germany.

2. Miles D. Landstuhl Outpatient Facility Makes Good on Promise to Wounded Warriors [news release]. American Forces Press Service; November 1, 2007.

3. Medical Transient Detachment, Landstuhl Regional Medical Center. *MTD Patient Policy Letters.* December 18, 2013.

4. Probus MC. *Analyzing the Requirement for a Deployed Warrior Medical Management Center Table of Distribution and Allowances at Landstuhl Regional Medical Center* [thesis]. Waco, TX: Baylor University; 2004.

BIBLIOGRAPHY

Cooper RA, Pasquina PF, Drach R, eds. *Warrior Transition Leader Medical Rehabilitation Handbook*. Fort Detrick, MD: Borden Institute; 2011.

Deployed Warrior Medical Management Center [news release]. Landstuhl, Germany: Landstuhl Regional Medical Center Public Affairs Office; July 2009.

Europe Regional Medical Command (ERMC). Fact Sheet—LRMC history: Landstuhl Regional Medical Center. Public Affairs Office. http://ermc. amedd.army.mil/landstuhl/factsheets/LRMCHistory.pdf. Accessed March 13, 2013.

Medical Transient Detachment Sidebar [news release no. 11]. Landstuhl, Germany: Landstuhl Regional Medical Center Public Affairs Office; April 22, 2008.

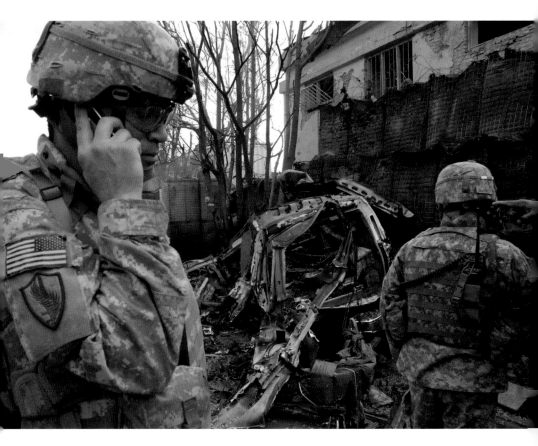

Members of the Camp Eggars Force Protection team assess the damage of an explosion near the gate on January 17, 2009. A vehicle-borne improvised explosive device (VBIED) exploded near the German Embassy and a US base in Kabul City, Afghanistan. The VBIED killed and wounded multinational personnel and damaged vehicles and nearby buildings.

Photographer: Technical Sergeant Brenda Nipper. Reproduced from: https://www. dvidshub.net/image/145118/vehicle-born-improvised-explosive-devide-explosion-kabul-city-afghanistan#.VuwVgzZf2pq.

CHAPTER FIVE

Traumatic Brain Injury

*It takes only seconds for an explosion to occur. It takes only those same
seconds for a life to be changed forever. This intersection of an instant in
time and a relentlessly chronic effect epitomizes the signature wound of the
Iraq and Afghanistan wars—traumatic brain injury.*

Since the United States went to war in Afghanistan in 2001, and Iraq in
2003, approximately 2 million US military personnel from every branch
have been deployed to the Middle East.[1] The lives of many of these service
members (SMs) and their families have been drastically impacted due to multiple
deployments, injuries, and death. Statistics and realities of this magnitude
have taken a grave toll on both the physical and psychological well-being of
our fighting soldiers. Traumatic brain injury (TBI) remains the most prevalent
injury among those who fought during Operation Enduring Freedom (OEF),
Operation Iraqi Freedom (OIF), and Operation New Dawn (OND).[2]

Improvised explosive devices (IEDs) are a lethal primary weapon of choice
used extensively against coalition forces in current warfare. This has significantly
changed the frontline milieu; death and injury are now measured more by
"cleverness of bombs rather than the accuracy of bullets."[3] The deleterious impact
of this type of warfare is further complicated by multiple deployments in which
soldiers are repeatedly exposed to ambushes by roadside bombs, IEDs, and the
effects from blast exposure.

Iraq is one of the most mine-infested nations in the world. Landmines have
been uncovered that date back as far as World War II, and since the early 1980s
this country has been involved in three wars. This ongoing strife meant that Iraqis
were learning continuously and extensively about explosives. The threat to US
military came from both the bomb and the bomb maker. By September 2003,
the design, construction, and technology of IEDs became more complex, and the
strategies behind using them became more organized and sophisticated.[4]

Exposure to a blast, and more significantly repetitive exposure, leaves a devastating neurological malady with a range of symptoms, such as memory problems, dizziness, sleeplessness, cognition problems, and mood changes. TBI occurs when a blow or jolt to the head or a penetrating head injury disrupts brain function and damages brain tissue.[5] When a blast such as that from an IED occurs, there are sudden changes in air pressure resulting in intense winds caused by the heat of the explosion and rapid movement of air molecules. Blast waves and powerful winds from explosions are strong enough to throw fragments, bodies, and even vehicles with tremendous force. These forces damage the brain, resulting in different levels of injury from mild (concussion) to severe and even penetrating injuries.[6]

Casualties treated for brain injuries were minimal during prior conflicts. In the Vietnam War, for example, mortality rates were greater than 75% for this type of injury, and survivors therefore comprised a small fraction of casualties treated in hospitals.[2] Improvements in helmets and Kevlar (DuPont, Wilmington, DE) body armor significantly decreased morbidities and mortalities in the current war because they better protect soldiers from bullets and fragments. However, even these improved helmets do not offer full protection because they do not completely cover the face, head, and neck. They cannot prevent closed-head trauma that occurs from blasts.[2]

TBI has been described as "one of the most complicated injuries to one of the most complicated parts of the body."[7] Symptoms range from mild to severe and may not necessarily correlate with the level of injury sustained. Physical and psychological impacts can be devastating and life altering at both personal and military levels. Therefore, development of the TBI program at Landstuhl Regional Medical Center (LRMC) was profoundly significant. Its mission is as follows:

> *The creation of a network of medical facilities working together to provide the required capability to screen, assess, treat, educate, follow-up, and conduct surveillance on all military mild and moderate TBI patients residing in the European theater.*[8]

BACKGROUND

The "community hospital" atmosphere of LRMC changed in 2001 when critical care needs escalated in conjunction with the beginning of the global war on terrorism. In 2005, the Trauma Team became aware of TBI as a commonly missed injury. This was not altogether surprising because the focus of care was placed on more obvious and acute injuries. Casualties were often passed through LRMC, and the initial diagnosis of TBI did not occur until patients were seen by medical providers in the continental United States (CONUS). The Trauma program at

LRMC then began collaborating with the Neurology Department and Behavioral Health Medicine to discuss why this diagnosis was being missed and to identify specific resource constraints at LRMC.

In March 2006, the Defense and Veterans Brain Injury Center (DVBIC) provided a Grand Rounds presentation to LRMC on TBI. The Trauma program and the Deployed Warrior Medical Management Center (DWMMC) subsequently collaborated on the development of a TBI tracking tool. In May 2006, the DWMMC staff began the initial identification of TBI through a formal, but limited, screening of combat casualties. They began collecting data from these screenings as well. In August 2006, the DWMMC issued a TBI screening policy statement that outlined formal roles and responsibilities for executing the TBI screening mission. A clinical management algorithm was implemented in November 2006 for those patients identified with mild TBI (also referred to as concussion). The Department of Defense (DoD) then modified evacuation protocols to route more severely affected patients to other centers with resources capable of providing sophisticated TBI rehabilitation. On March 23, 2007, the Assistant Secretary of Defense issued a memorandum outlining the consolidation of TBI initiatives in the DoD under the Deputy Assistant Secretary of Defense for Force Health Protection and Readiness.[9] The US Army Medical Research and Materiel Command would coordinate all DoD research related to TBI. This was important because Congress wanted the US Army to take on the role of Executive Agent for TBI. DVBIC was designated as the single office responsible for the consolidation of all TBI-related incidence and prevalence information collected by all services. DVBIC had existed for many years and consisted of subject matter experts on TBI.

In October 2007, the Office of The Surgeon General (OTSG) distributed a memorandum outlining requirements for TBI certification for all Army military medical treatment facilities (MTFs) and a gap analysis to compare the present performance with future desired outcomes.[10,11] Information gained from these documents would be the Army's first attempt to develop and then provide a standardized approach to creating an organizational structure to build TBI programs.

In April 2008, the US Army Medical Command Headquarters issued Operations Order 08-39, *The Army Medical Command Traumatic Brain Injury (TBI) Action Plan*, which outlined additional requirements needed for the establishment of TBI treatment capabilities at all Army MTFs.[12] In mid-2008, the DWMMC passed complete responsibility for all TBI screenings of inpatient and outpatient OIF/OEF SMs to the Trauma program.

The OTSG memorandum and the gap analysis identified a lack of equipment, space, financial resources, and personnel to staff a TBI program at LRMC. Clinicians from Sterling Medical Corporation, Inc (a healthcare staffing

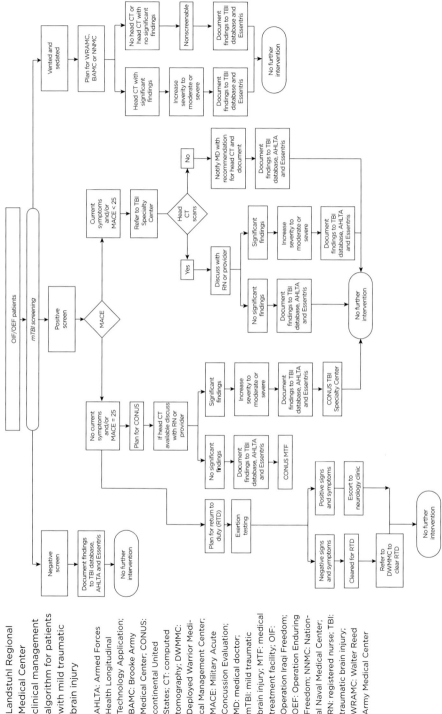

Landstuhl Regional Medical Center clinical management algorithm for patients with mild traumatic brain injury

AHLTA: Armed Forces Health Longitudinal Technology Application; BAMC: Brooke Army Medical Center; CONUS: continental United States; CT: computed tomography; DWMMC: Deployed Warrior Medical Management Center; MACE: Military Acute Concussion Evaluation; MD: medical doctor; mTBI: mild traumatic brain injury; MTF: medical treatment facility; OIF: Operation Iraqi Freedom; OEF: Operation Enduring Freedom; NNMC: National Naval Medical Center; RN: registered nurse; TBI: traumatic brain injury; WRAMC: Walter Reed Army Medical Center organization in Cincinnati, OH), were then contracted and arrived in Germany in December 2008. It was believed that using contract clinicians would reduce risk and provide the greatest flexibility to the Army as it developed TBI programs across the nation and overseas. Unfortunately, the timing and order of arrival of resources were not optimal. In ideal circumstances, resources such as space and equipment are obtained prior to the arrival of clinical staff. Unfortunately, the exact opposite occurred. Personnel showed up first, which created a tremendous challenge in finding a workspace for them within the existing hospital structure. In a few cases, such as speech and language pathology, the existing clinic had an extra room and desks to accommodate the two new clinicians. However, this was not the norm. The TBI program was given some limited space in a newly renovated wing of the hospital; however, this appointed space came without equipment or furniture.

Developing the infrastructure, understanding resource and budget processes, and navigating through layers of bureaucracy were essential skills needed to meet the OTSG requirements. These are skills that are not known to most clinicians. The critical need for a program manager was, therefore, quite apparent. The position was finally filled in March 2009 and proved vital to the success of meeting the OTSG requirements for establishing a TBI program.

In May 2009, the TBI Screening Team was officially transferred from the Trauma program to the TBI program under the Department of Neurology. The Intensive Rehabilitation Program piloted its first cohort in August 2009 with a dedicated TBI Rehabilitation Center building opening in November 2010. Beginning that month, the LRMC TBI program utilized a variety of specialists to responsibly serve the European TBI patient population. This continues to be the current practice. Although the drawdown in Iraq and Afghanistan has resulted in decreased patient encounters it has not diminished the requirement to provide key program elements nor the goal of addressing the complex and multidisciplinary needs of TBI patients.

IMPLEMENTATION METHODS

Leadership Staffing

Leadership staffing consists of the following personnel:
- medical director (physiatrist),
- program manager,
- noncommissioned officer in charge (NCOIC), and
- team leaders.

Each of the TBI program elements has an assigned team leader who reports to the medical director on clinical matters and to the program manager for nonclinical issues.

Program Elements

The TBI program is composed of nine program elements:

1. TBI Screening,
2. Initial Evaluation/Treatment Planning,
3. Case Management,
4. TBI Rehabilitation,
5. Research,
6. Data/ANAM (Automated Neuropsychological Assessment Metrics) Management,
7. Education,
8. Telehealth, and
9. Clinical/Business Operations.

Traumatic Brain Injury Screening

The TBI Screening Team consists of the following:

- one registered nurse (RN) team leader,
- two RN nurse screeners,
- two licensed practical nurse (LPN) screeners, and
- one social services assistant.

The Screening Team's mission is to ensure that all military personnel, civilians (DoD and contractors), and coalition military personnel medevaced from the theater of operation for OND/OEF undergo TBI screening before returning to CONUS or return to duty (RTD). OND/OEF refers to those patients who are medevaced from Iraq, Afghanistan, the Horn of Africa (Djibouti), Kuwait, Qatar, and Dubai. In addition, Kosovo and Bosnia fall under the Joint Program Management Guardian and are included under the OND/OEF umbrella.

The initial screening tool is a self-reporting survey administered to all OND/OEF patients medevaced to LRMC. The three key components of this screening questionnaire include (1) type of TBI exposure (eg, blast, vehicle collision, fall), (2) immediate symptoms following the event (eg, loss of consciousness, confusion, no recollection), and (3) symptoms experienced since the event (eg, headache, dizziness, memory loss).[13] All patients are given an individual appointment with a TBI Screening Team member that lasts between 5 and 45 minutes, depending on whether there are indicators of a possible TBI event. Any patient who screens positive (with or without symptoms) is subsequently assessed using the DVBIC's Military Acute Concussion Evaluation (MACE).[13] This document is used to gauge the severity of symptoms and cognitive deficits. The questionnaire consists of three components:

Landstuhl Regional Medical Center patient screening questionnaire for traumatic brain injury

LRMC Traumatic Brain Injury Program
Patient Screening Questionnaire
(version 4.14.08)

DATE and TIME of Screening (DD-MMM-YYYY)	NAME (Last, First)		SSN	DOB (DD-MMM-YYYY)	Home Date of Record	Duty Station
- - [:]			- -	- -		

Age	Gender	Pt Status	Date of Admission/Arrival (DD-MMM-YYYY)	Time of Admission	Pt. Location		Patient Contact (CONUS ph#)
	M / F	Out / In			ICU / 8D / 9C / 10C / 10D / 13D/ 14D		

Branch (Circle one)	Service Status (circle one)	Rank/Pay Grade	Originating (circle one)
Army / AF / Marine / Navy / Coalition:_____ / Civilian	AD / RES / NG / CIV		OIF / OEF / OTHER
Planned destination (Circle one) Other:____ Theater / CONUS / Local / OCONUS / UNK	Primary diagnosis: NBI BI DNBI (Circle one)		Data entry person

How many times have you been deployed (OIF/ OEF) ? _____   # of months on Current Deployment _____

Questions 1 & 2 must be COMPLETED. If there are no positive results, please check "None of the above".

1. During this deployment, did you experience any of the following events?
(Please check all that apply and for each YES, note the number of each episode)

A. O Blast   #____
(IED, RPG, Landmine, Grenades, etc.)

D. O Bullet wound   #____
(above the shoulders)

F. O Fragment wound   #____
(above the shoulders)

B. O Fall   #____
(striking head)

E. O Vehicular crashes   #____
(any vehicle including aircraft)

G. O None of the Above

C. O Other Significant contact with blunt object
(above the shoulders)   Describe:

2. If you answered Yes to Question #1, did you experience any of these symptoms IMMEDIATELY afterwards?
(Please check all that apply)

O LOC (Knocked out) for less than 1 minute

O LOC for greater than 1 hour.

O Being dazed, confused, or "seeing stars" (feeling disconnected from yourself or the environment)

O LOC from 1 to 30 minutes.

O Not remembering the injury

O None of the Above

O LOC from 31 minutes up to 1 hour.

If your answer to 1 is "None of the Above" ....Skip to Question #8

3. If you answered POSITIVELY to question 2., what was the date of your injury.
Enter answer using the following format 'dd mmm yyyy' If unsure of exact date use the 1st of the month
Circle letter of the corresponding event   A   B   C   D   E   F   (DD-MMM-YYYY)

Primary Injury Event History:

What was your estimated distance from the blast? (in meters)
If you were in a vehicle during the injury event, what was the type of vehicle?
If you were in a vehicle during the injury event, what was your position in the vehicle?

4. If you answered POSITIVELY to question #2, were you wearing protective gear at the time of the injury?   O YES   O NO

5. If you answered POSITIVELY to question #2. what protective gear were you wearing? (check all that apply)

O Kevlar Helmet
O IBA Groin protector
O IBA Side plates
O Other

O IBA Vest
O IBA Front Armor Plate
O Eye Protection
O Gloves

O IBA Collar
O IBA Back Armor Plate
O Hearing Protection
O IOTV

LRMC TBI Screening Form.doc

Courtesy of the Landstuhl Regional Medical Center Traumatic Brain Injury Program.

1. history of injury and symptoms,
2. cognitive screen with score, and
3. screening neurological examination.

All patients with an abnormal MACE score (symptomatic and asymptomatic) are referred to a neurologist for a more comprehensive evaluation and possible radiographic imaging with either computed tomography (CT) or magnetic resonance imaging (MRI) scans.[13]

The screening at LRMC is only an initial assessment; 85% of the patients medevaced from downrange continue to CONUS within 72 hours of arriving at LRMC.

Initial Evaluation/Treatment Planning

The Initial Evaluation/Treatment Planning Team consists of a neurologist and a nurse practitioner. Both are under the supervision of the program medical director.

SMs who have had a potential TBI event and who are currently having symptoms associated with that event (termed positive symptomatic) are referred to the neurology clinic to receive clinical confirmation of the TBI diagnosis. A comprehensive neurological examination may reveal abnormalities of the cranial nerves, postural stability/vestibular system, and visual function.

SMs who had a potential TBI event, who are not currently having symptoms associated with that event (termed positive asymptomatic), and who are requesting an RTD are referred to the neurology clinic to confirm the diagnosis and undergo an exertion test prior to clearance for RTD. An exertion test raises the heart rate of a patient for a set period of time to determine if TBI-related symptoms return. No patient screened positive asymptomatic can RTD unless he or she undergoes the exertion test and has a MACE score greater than or equal to 25.[13]

SMs who had a potential TBI event, who are not currently having symptoms associated with that event (positive asymptomatic), and who are not requesting RTD are free to continue with all other appointments and processing. No further TBI action is required for these SMs at LRMC, except for documentation and education.

The initial TBI screening, exertional testing results, and TBI evaluations are documented in the inpatient and outpatient medical records of all patients evacuated through LRMC. Data are entered into the TBI database, and this information is subsequently available to healthcare providers in CONUS.

Case Management

The Case Management (CM) Team consists of three RN case managers. Nurse CM is a collaborative process of assessment, planning, facilitation, care coordination, evaluation, and advocacy to meet the comprehensive healthcare needs of an individual or family.

Nurse case managers act as liaisons between the patient, healthcare providers, commanders, and community resources to achieve high-quality, patient-centered, cost-effective outcomes with an emphasis on health promotion, maintenance, education, and risk prevention.

TBI Evaluation: A sample of the assessment used to screen for traumatic brain injury known as MACE (Military Acute Concussion Evaluation). The test has a possible 30 points. Patients without concussions average a score of 28. Scores below 25 indicate a possible diagnosis of TBI.

IMMEDIATE MEMORY: 15 points (1 point for each correct answer over three trials)
A test giver will say five random words and ask a patient to repeat them in any order. Test giver and patient repeat this two more times for a total of three trials.

ORIENTATION: 5 points (1 point for each)
Patients are given five time and date questions.

CONCENTRATION: 5 points (1 point for each)
Patients are told a string of numbers and asked to recall the numbers in reverse order. The number strings range from three to six digits in length. Then patients are asked to recite the months of the year in reverse order.

DELAYED RECALL: 5 points (1 point for each)
Without the test giver repeating the same five words from the immediate memory portion, patients are asked to recall the five words from the first portion of the test.

Source: Defense and Veterans Brain Injury Center, Silver Spring, MD.
For the complete version of the MACE screening, see http://www.pdhealth.mil/downloads/MACE.pdf.

The TBI nurse case manager coordinates TBI referrals, ensures that all SMs receive individualized treatment plans, and provides for comprehensive continuity of care for all SMs identified as potential TBI patients. Case managers work in three areas:
1. screening-intake and referral,
2. intensive rehabilitation, and
3. follow-up.

Traumatic Brain Injury Rehabilitation

The TBI Rehabilitation Team consists of a strong interdisciplinary team of providers from the following disciplines: neurology, primary care, physiatry, physical therapy, occupational therapy, speech language pathology, behavioral health, optometry, audiology, pain management, vocational rehabilitation counseling, and the Chaplain's Office. Additional specialists are consulted as needed.

The Intensive Rehabilitation Program at LRMC, known as "Synapse," is currently for USAREUR (US Army Europe) soldiers and their dependents whose needs cannot be met at their home station TBI centers for reasons such as increasing symptoms, unavailability of specialists, and recommendations of local TBI treatment teams. The purpose of the program is to coordinate the care and integration of medical services and therapeutic resources that are critical to the SMs receiving rehabilitation for concussion care. The program eliminates the need for

Synapse Group Therapies: An example of the types of programs, interventions, and specialists involved in the Synapse Intensive Rehabilitation Program. Each patient has an individual treatment plan based on his or her particular needs as determined by the evaluation and clinical team. The Synapse Treatment Team is happy to involve family members or significant others in the program, with consent. Team members can help educate family members regarding relevant symptoms, therapy, progress, and outcomes. This can be done in-person or by telephone.

MORNING GROUP: The day begins with a review of the daily schedule and participation in short activities to get focused. Patients meet briefly with their case manager and the occupational therapist to organize their scheduled treatments.

COGNITIVE GAME GROUP: The Cognitive Gaming group is designed to provide an opportunity to practice cognitive skills in a fun and interactive environment. The group is facilitated by a speech-language pathologist and an occupational therapist. A variety of group, solo, and two-player games are provided that specifically challenge skills, such as: working memory, problem-solving, planning, creative thinking, visual spatial skills, and fast-paced attention. Participation will be part of a therapy plan and tracked as therapy goals. Group members who are not being seen for cognitive skills development are welcome to participate as space permits.

CONDITIONING & STRENGTH TRAINING: Patients participate in a physical therapy-directed approach to improving circulation, flexibility, and neuromuscular function. This enhances other aspects of treatment by providing opportunities to improve sleep and concentration, and decrease stress and tension headaches.

VOCATIONAL EDUCATION GROUP: This group focuses on goal setting, and establishing objectives for either successful reintegration into work and education or preparation for transition. This group is co-facilitated by individuals who have experienced traumatic brain injury and the group is focused on cognitive reframing to support recovery, quality of life, and personal goals.

MINDFULNESS/RELAXATION: A variety of activities will be utilized to increase mental and emotional focus, a sense of relaxation, and regulation of the nervous system.

PSYCHOEDUCATIONAL/OCCUPATIONAL GROUP: A variety of educational resources and small group options are available to the patient to address specific vocational aspects of his or her rehabilitation as well as provide the patient with educational opportunities to increase awareness and understanding of recovery from concussion.

Source: Landstuhl Regional Medical Center Traumatic Brain Injury Program.

local SMs and those from downrange who require short-term outpatient care for TBI-related symptoms (eg, headaches, balance problems) from having to navigate multiple clinics at LRMC. Local patients needing care beyond the scope of their stationed health clinic can travel to LRMC for more intensive treatment, including the Synapse program. This intensive intervention at LRMC meets the individual needs of each SM, and can be for a few weeks or as long as 8 weeks based on the unique symptom presentation.

The interdisciplinary team first evaluates TBI patients using a multidiscipline assessment process to determine if they meet the appropriate criteria for intensive rehabilitation. If their needs require this level of intervention, they are accepted into the Synapse program and an interdisciplinary treatment plan is developed and reviewed with the patient. Based on individual needs, daily intensive therapy is scheduled that includes a combination of one-on-one and group treatment sessions. For those individuals who do not require the level of intense rehabilitation offered through Synapse, appropriate recommendations are made.

The primary mission of the Rehabilitation Team is to maximize the quality of life and recovery of function for all TBI patients referred to LRMC. The assessment for comorbidities is especially critical given the circumstances under which the injuries have occurred. The Synapse program works closely with the LRMC Evolutions program, a comprehensive day treatment approach to treating posttraumatic stress disorder (PTSD). If a patient experiences complex symptoms related to PTSD, the team may recommend that the individual attend the Evolutions program. For problematic but less intense trauma-based treatment needs, patients may receive individual or group psychotherapy with behavioral health providers within the Synapse program.

It is also incumbent upon the team to determine the ability of the patient to RTD and to then facilitate that goal. The team meets weekly to ensure that all patients are receiving appropriate treatment plans, monitor progress, review goals, and formulate a comprehensive discharge plan. They also work closely with command to communicate patient progress. If it seems likely the SM will RTD, the team also works with command to review job function and performance, and tailors treatment toward addressing specific job capacities needed for that SM to function within his or her military occupational specialty. Educating SMs and their families about their recovery, and how to cope with all the factors related to TBI, is a vital part of the program. Treatment plans are developed at discharge, and follow-up services can often be implemented via telemedicine and home therapy programs, or with local providers at the patient's home base of record.

Research

The Research Team consists of a research coordinator who is a licensed rehabilitative psychologist.

The TBI research coordinator works with the entire research community at LRMC to facilitate research activities, provides subject matter expertise on TBI-related research, and manages the programmatic coordination of all TBI research trials. Examples of proposed projects include the following:

Project 1:   Secondary Data Analysis Trial
Purpose: To review 2010 TBI screening database for trajectory of recovery and
               care models.

Project 2:   Banyan Biomarkers Trial
Purpose: Pilot study ($N = 30$) on acute, subacute, and chronic serum
               biomarkers for TBI.

Project 3:   Visual-Ocular Motor Trial
Purpose: To review visual-ocular motor vision therapy provided to 500 soldiers
               in 2008 to model care recovery and benefit from therapy.

Project 4:   TBI Outcome Measures
Purpose: To explore common outcome measures for mild TBI assessment,
               evaluation, and treatment.

Project 5:   TBI Trial: ANAM vs ImPACT (Immediate Post-Concussion
               Assessment and Cognitive Testing)
Purpose: To evaluate efficacy of various automated neuropsychological
               assessment metrics.

Project 6:   RU486 Trial
Purpose: To assess the efficacy of RU486 (mifepristone) in the treatment of
               combat-related PTSD.

Project 7:   Clinical Trials Enterprise
Purpose: To evaluate clinical trial enterprise markers in military members.

Project 8:   ADVAB/WTAR (Armed Services Vocational Aptitude Battery/
               Wechsler Test of Adult Reading) Trial
Purpose: To demonstrate the association between ADVAB general technical
               scores and WTAR.

Project 9:   TBI Education Trial
Purpose: To examine the efficacy of TBI education on improving recovery and
               rehabilitation outcomes in military patients.

Project 10:   Natural History Trial
Purpose: To examine the trajectory of recovery from mild TBI in military
               soldiers.

Data/Automated Neuropsychological Assessment Metrics Management

The Data/ANAM Team consists of a data management specialist (who is in charge of the team), two trained ANAM testing facilitators at each military MTF, and five ANAM psychology technicians strategically placed across the Europe Regional Medical Command (ERMC) area of responsibility.

In May 2008, the Assistant Secretary of Defense (Health Affairs Office) issued a memorandum mandating that all SMs receive a predeployment computerized neurocognitive assessment using the ANAM.[14] The purpose of the test was to establish baseline information of brain function. In the event that the SM sustained a TBI, the test could then be retaken and the results compared with the original to monitor any changes in cognitive function. The ANAM is a computer program that detects speed and accuracy of attention, memory, and reaction time. Performance is measured through responses provided on a computer, and the test takes about 20 minutes to complete.[15] The DVBIC has been designated as the office of responsibility for this DoD program, referred to as the Neurocognitive Assessment Tool Program.

The primary mission is to ensure that the ANAM program is fully coordinated across ERMC. Prior to deployment, ERMC incorporates baseline ANAM testing results for all deploying soldiers into either soldier readiness processing, periodic health assessment, or predeployment processing, and then supports postinjury ANAM testing when clinically indicated and ordered by a medical provider.

The data management specialist is responsible for administrative control of the TBI Screening Access Database and development of a TBI Clinical Outcomes Database.

Education

The framework of the rehabilitative program is the belief that a positive course of recovery from any degree of a TBI begins and ends with education, which is therefore mandatory for SMs, beneficiaries, and retirees. In addition, TBI education is given to TBI providers and staff, other nonspecific hospital and clinic providers and staff, regular line units, and other community organizations.

In-service educational briefings on the screening process used for TBI patients are given on a monthly basis for both new employee orientation and the Department of Nursing orientation. A member of the TBI Screening Team provides an overview of TBI at both briefings and also quarterly to the hospital wards, outpatient clinics, and outlying Army health clinics. In addition, the TBI screeners give DVBIC-approved verbal and written TBI educational information to patients who have a positive result for concussion on their screen. Providers caring for the TBI-identified patient will continue the education process by affirming the expected recovery and providing an individualized plan of care.

A full-time RN education coordinator is available to facilitate and coordinate educational activities for local TBI patients, family members, commands, providers, and the community. A midlevel provider (eg, a nurse practitioner), with experience in treating patients who have sustained a TBI, coordinates educational activities targeted specifically to providers across the ERMC. This training and education include face-to-face and videoteleconference briefings, proctorships, conference lectures, and electronic information dissemination.

Telehealth

All military personnel, civilians (DoD and contractors), and coalition military personnel who are evaluated by the interdisciplinary team for the TBI Intensive Rehabilitation Program are eligible to receive follow-up rehabilitative care through the use of telehealth resources and videoteleconferencing. This telehealth capability has been instrumental in reducing travel costs for patients spread across the European region and also in reducing time away from the workplace.

Clinical/Business Operations

Clinical/business operations for the TBI program is led by the TBI NCOIC. The NCOIC serves as the supervisor for three medical support assistants (a GS-04 position) and one administrative assistant (a GS-06 position).

Clinical operations encompass all of the duties and responsibilities that facilitate day-to-day patient care and facility management. These include, but are not limited to, the following:

- front desk management;
- safety and hazardous material training;
- infectious control;
- information management, performance management, and representative management;
- medical equipment and supply chain management;
- property and inventory management; and
- facilities and equipment maintenance management.

Business operations encompass the following duties and responsibilities:

- financial management,
- personnel status management,
- timekeeping,
- key control management,
- patient/visitor control, and
- reports and data analysis.

ADDITIONAL TRACKING TOOLS

- *TBI Screening Database.* This is a Microsoft Access-based database that stores all TBI screening data collected by the TBI Screening Team. Because of HIPPA (Health Insurance Portability and Accountability Act) regulations, this database is restricted, and information is not available to the public.
- *Intensive Rehabilitation One-Note CM Files.* This is an interdisciplinary, HIPAA-secure, collaborative, shared database that assists case managers and providers in managing intensive rehabilitation planning and treatment progress.

LESSONS LEARNED

Military hospitals experience the stark reality of increased patient volume and more serious injuries during any sort of armed conflict. The high rate of TBI and blast-related concussion events resulting from current combat operations directly impacts the health and safety of individual SMs, and subsequently the level of unit readiness and troop retention. The impact of TBI has been felt within each branch of the service and throughout both the DoD and the Department of Veterans Affairs healthcare systems.

The creation of the TBI program at LRMC was a paramount contribution to the overall care of wounded warriors impacted by this diagnosis. The importance of early identification and assessment of TBI symptoms facilitated patient care, provider communication, and appropriate rehabilitative intervention. Although creating the clinical structure to address patient needs was an integral piece of the program, building and operating an environment to effectively work in was the far greater challenge. This fully integrated interdisciplinary team approach to TBI treatment and management continues to be an important mission of LRMC.

Successes

- *Traumatic brain injury screening.* Since the initiation of the TBI database in March 2006, more than 43,000 TBI screenings have been conducted at LRMC and more than 8,500 positive screens have been identified, which likely would have gone undetected without this program. The creation of a dedicated TBI Screening Team paid great dividends toward workload allocation and early identification of TBI in those patients with obvious head injuries, and even more so in those patients with no external indications.
- *Traumatic brain injury encounters.* TBI encounters are documented with an ICD-10-CM (*International Classification of Diseases, 10th Revision, Clinical Modification*) diagnosis code of V15.52, "Personal

History of TBI." From October 2009 to September 2012, LRMC staff documented more than 30,000 TBI specific encounters.

- *Traumatic brain injury rehabilitation.* Since the start of the TBI Intensive Rehabilitation Program in August 2009, LRMC has managed more than 500 SMs for symptoms associated with a TBI event. By fiscal year 2011, the program had attained a 65% RTD rate. At an estimated $250,000 invested training cost per SM, this program resulted in cost avoidance to the US Army in excess of $79.9 million.[16]

- *Research.* Since the initiation of the TBI database in March 2006, a number of research trials and projects were conducted that provided pertinent information affecting clinical outcomes. The role of the TBI research coordinator was especially valuable to LRMC participation in national protocols because a tremendous amount of time is needed to ensure that trial development, approval, and execution occur. TBI research must continue to move forward, and the local military hospital needs to be a vital partner in the process.

- *Education.* Educating SMs and their support systems on engaging in their own recovery and considering factors in their lives that influence a positive course of rehabilitation has been a vital component to the success of the TBI program, and for discharge and follow-up planning. A positive course of recovery from brain injury begins and ends with education. Every component of LRMC's intensive program emphasizes the importance of a holistic and dynamic recovery process. Awareness and understanding of the expected course of recovery from brain injury creates empowerment, which is how patients rebuild a sense of normalcy and develop self-efficacy.

- *Award.* The Surgeon General and the chief of the Army Medical Department Civilian Corps created the Wolf Pack Award to recognize exceptional teamwork by an integrated group of military and civilian team members focused on excellence in support of Army Medicine. In the first quarter of fiscal year 2012, the TBI team at LRMC was the recipient of the Wolf Pack Award.

Challenges

- *Maintaining the mission.* Assessing and treating TBI-related symptoms is a core mission of the Army. Maintaining this focus will require continued vigilance in the areas of TBI care, research, education, and outreach. Although recent attention has been intensively focused on combat-related TBI, it should be noted that the majority of TBI-related injuries are non–combat-related. Many routine operational and training activities in the military are physically demanding and even potentially dangerous. TBI incidents also occur in garrison during daily activities. SMs enjoy exciting leisure activities: they ride motorcycles, climb mountains, and parachute from planes for recreation. Although both the training and recreational activities are expected for SMs and contribute to a positive quality of life, they also can increase the risk for TBI.

- *Reintegration.* The challenges faced by TBI patients and their families are enormous. Brain injuries can affect motor, sensory, cognitive, and behavioral functioning. SMs who have sustained a TBI may have difficulty returning to work, school, and family life, or engaging in activities enjoyed prior to injury. The high number of wounded warriors with TBI has highlighted and reinforced the need for various types of support as they attempt to reintegrate. Both garrison leaders and the general community need to reach out and help soldiers reintegrate with families, friends, work, and activities. It is not uncommon for SMs with TBI to also experience PTSD. Encouraging those SMs to ask for help when they are struggling so that appropriate interventions can be made is paramount to their recovery and family cohesiveness. Community support plays a vital role in the rehabilitative continuum of care.

- *Model of care.* For the majority of wounded SMs, TBI (typically mild) was only one diagnosis of many. Identifying and treating comorbidities in a coordinated fashion has been crucial for this population. Future programs would benefit by focusing on combat rehabilitation, as opposed to a single diagnosis-driven rehabilitation. By emphasizing function and identifying all diagnoses that are impacting it, the patient's quality of life becomes the central coordinating influence around which care is provided. This patient-centered and patient-directed care model helps patients reestablish a quality of life that is meaningful and personally relevant.

ACKNOWLEDGMENTS

The authors thank David Williams and LTC Megumi Vogt, US Army.

REFERENCES

1. Hosek J. *How Is Deployment to Iraq and Afghanistan Affecting U.S. Service Members and Their Families? An Overview of Early RAND Research on the Topic.* Santa Monica, CA: RAND Corporation; 2011. http://www.rand.org/pubs/occasional_papers/OP316. Accessed July 29, 2015.

2. Okie S. Traumatic brain injury in the war zone. *N Engl J Med.* 2005;352: 2043–2047.

3. Dao J. Afghan war's buried bombs put risk in every step. *New York Times.* July 15, 2009.

4. McFate M. Iraq: the social context of IEDS. *Mil Rev.* 2005;May–June: 37–40.

5. National Institute of Neurologic Disorders and Stroke. NINDS traumatic brain injury information page. http://www.ninds.nih.gov/disorders/tbi/tbi.htm Accessed June 22, 2015.

6. Hicks R, Fertig S, Desrocher R, Koroshetz W, Pancrazio J. Neurologic effects of blast injury. *J Trauma.* 2010;68(5):1257–1263.

7. Alvarez L. War veterans' concussions are often overlooked. *New York Times.* August 25, 2008.

8. Landstuhl Regional Medical Center Public Affairs Office. *Fact Sheet: Traumatic Brain Injury.* Landstuhl, Germany: LRMC PAO; 2013.

9. Winkenwerder W. *Consolidation of Traumatic Brain Injury Initiatives in the Department of Defense.* Washington, DC: Assistant Secretary of Defense, Health Affairs. Memorandum to the Assistant Secretary of the Army, Assistant Secretary of the Navy, Assistant Secretary of the Air Force, Surgeon General of the Army, Surgeon General of the Navy, and Surgeon General of the Air Force; March 23, 2007.

10. Casscells SW. *Traumatic Brain Injury: Definition and Reporting.* Washington, DC: Assistant Secretary of Defense, Health Affairs. Memorandum to the Assistant Secretary of the Army, Assistant Secretary of the Navy, and Assistant Secretary of the Air Force; October 1, 2007.

11. US Army Combined Arms Center. *Army Operational Knowledge Management: KM Gap Analysis.* Fort Leavenworth, KS: USACAC; 2013.

12. Army Medical Command Headquarters. *The Army Medical Command Traumatic Brain Injury (TBI) Action Plan (AP).* Fort Sam Houston, TX: MEDCOM; 2008. Operations Order 08-39.

13. Dempsey KE, Dorlac WC, Martin K, et al. Landstuhl Regional Medical Center: traumatic brain injury screening program. *J Trauma Nurs.* 2009;16(1):6–12.

14. Casscells SW. *Baseline Pre-deployment Neurocognitive Functional Assessment— Interim Guidance.* Washington, DC: Memorandum to the Assistant Secretary of the Army, Assistant Secretary of the Navy, and Assistant Secretary of the Air Force; May 28, 2008.

15. Defense Centers of Excellence for Psychological Health and Brain Injury. *Fact Sheet: Automated Neuropsychological Assessment Metrics Management (ANAM).* Silver Spring, MD: DCoE; Summer 2012.

16. Statistics provided by Williams D, Vogt M, Landstuhl Regional Medical Center Traumatic Brain Injury Program, February 2013.

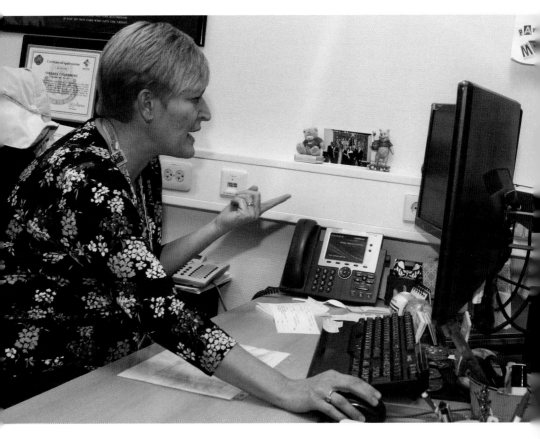

Another busy day on the job for Shelley Ohlendorf,
Supervisor, Wounded Warrior Finance Office.

Photograph courtesy of the Public Affairs Office,
Landstuhl Regional Medical Center.

CHAPTER SIX

Wounded Warrior Finance Office

"Success is the sum of small efforts, repeated day in and day out."

— ROBERT COLLIER

---

*From point of arrival at LRMC, to point of designated departure,
the Wounded Warrior Pay Office supports each soldier through every step
of this process. The combination of professional financial support, vigilant
monitoring, and premier customer service has eliminated untold financial
stress for these wounded warriors and their families.
This office is the quintessential example of "mission accomplished!"
All team members see this unique job opportunity as a life-changing,
rewarding honor serving our nation's heroes.*

First Sergeant Shelley Ohlendorf worked in the finance office during her deploy-ment to Iraq. Unbeknownst to her at the time, this experience was the segue to her future position at Landstuhl Regional Medical Center (LRMC). She retired from the military after 26 years of service and remained in Germany with her husband and sons. It was the first time in her life she stayed at home and did not work. Eventually, Shelley became restless; she needed a new purpose. By August 2007, the Wounded Warrior Pay Management Team at LRMC needed a supervisor, and they hired her for the position. The team had been established to prevent debts for combat zone entitlements for injured or sick soldiers evacuated from downrange.

Battle-injured soldiers face daunting challenges physically, emotionally, and financially. Many of them undergo multiple surgeries followed by months of physical rehabilitation. Some soldiers are unable to return to duty or, worse yet, to their military careers. Such injuries can be life-altering, calling for a reassessment of goals and an adjustment to physical limitations.

The mission of the Wounded Warrior Pay Management Team is as follows: *To improve the accuracy and the timeliness of pay to Wounded Warriors and their*

Finding New Purpose

She was known as "Mama O" to her battalion in Balad, Iraq. Deployed in 2003, First Sergeant Shelley Ohlendorf was no stranger to hard work, hard conditions, danger, or commitment to the mission. She remembers no running water, no electricity, and washing her laundry in a trash bag. She was the protective, but tough, First Sergeant yelling to her unit at any hour of the night "to get to the bunkers" with the first sounds of exploding mortars, watching the night air enveloped in suffocating clouds of black smoke. To this day, Shelley cringes at the sound of fireworks and avoids claustrophobic places. Mama O earned her nickname because she was also a caring mother figure—nurturing, listening, and looking to keep sagging spirits high. Undaunted by limited resources, she used a one-burner Coleman stove to make Mickey Mouse pancakes for her soldiers on Christmas morning in Balad. Shelley was a mother of two boys herself. She understood that the simplest things can make a difference.

Wanting to learn more, Shelley remembers her first visit to LRMC. She was observing the team she would soon lead, and watched as the AMBUS (ambulance bus) pulled to the front of the hospital to offload sick and injured soldiers. She watched the stretchers come down off the bus, intensive care patients the first priority. All Shelley could see was tubing and equipment; not the patient nor the person with him who had helped keep him alive. She remembers being glad it was raining because no one could see the tears in her eyes. Shelley Ohlendorf knew she wanted to be part of this team; she wanted to ease this suffering in some capacity. This was the right thing to do. "Mama O" had found her new purpose.

families and to ensure the critical human dimension of pay support (face-to-face contact to educate the customer) occurs at all critical patient flow locations.[1]

BACKGROUND

When soldiers are injured and medically evacuated, they are quickly whisked off for appropriate care, thus leaving their units before their mobilization period officially ends. A soldier's pay status is dependent on his or her status or location. Prior to 2005, the lack of a centralized automated data system meant that a soldier's duty status was not automatically updated when he or she was medically evacuated. Without the proper input of changes in wounded warrior status, finance battalions were not receiving the necessary substantiating documents, and appropriate pay changes were therefore not made. This led to pay-related problems, including in some cases substantial debt, which caused undue stress for the soldiers and their families.

In tracing the problem backward, it became apparent that the lack of a centralized patient tracking system was the pivotal underlying issue responsible for these erroneous overpayments. This essential realization then led to the establishment of a Senior Non-Commissioned Officer (NCO) Patient Tracking Team by the US Army Europe (USAREUR) G1 (personnel office) at LRMC because it was the prime location for medevaced (medical evacuation) missions. The team was responsible for 100% accountability of all warriors medevaced *to* LRMC and for providing updates on those that departed *from* LRMC either for return to their units or for transfer to CONUS (continental United States) for continued care. The team generated daily Casualty Information Center reports to account for these Army MEDEVAC soldiers. Shortly after, a decision was made to also involve finance soldiers; trained military personnel with specialization in military pay, travel pay, resource management, accounting, etc. This was an essential support supplement because Europe-based finance units were already on rotational deployments to theater to support deployed units and the needs at LRMC demanded consistency. The finance soldiers in turn coordinated with the Patient Tracking Team and LRMC medical staff to provide the necessary support needed for the medevaced soldiers.

In October 2005, a wounded warrior pay mission was implemented as a preventive measure to minimize overpayment of combat zone entitlements by the US government to wounded warriors. At this point, there was growing realization of soldiers incurring debt from overpayments of continuing combat zone entitlements if they were not accounted for. The two to three Army finance soldiers assigned from the battalions under the 266th Finance Command were now the first official finance team at LRMC, and they were assigned to meet with each wounded warrior. The goal was to prevent debt by ensuring accountability for those warriors being medevaced from theater, verifying inpatient or outpatient status, and reporting who was being transferred to CONUS for further medical care. The Defense Finance and Accounting Services (DFAS) developed the Wounded in Action (WIA) database in June 2005, and LRMC became the "hub of the wheel" for the Army-wide program.[2]

Challenges arose, however, as the initial Wounded Warrior Finance Team worked with minimal resources. Standard operating procedures had yet to be created to handle this unique organization. Efforts were aimed at accounting for medevaced soldiers, providing needed finance support, answering pay-related inquiries, and working an expedited debt remission process if overpayments occurred. Young warriors in particular needed help in navigating through the system because many had never been in a hospital and were overwhelmed by the entire experience. These soldiers were unsure if they were financially responsible for their medical bills and if they had to pay for their equipment that was lost or damaged during the attack that injured them. To further complicate the issues at hand, the wounded warrior finance team was not yet a *full-time* mission. In fact, it was more of an intermittent mission as the team juggled supporting other finance missions throughout Europe and training for their own deployments. Minimal staff working with minimal office equipment found it increasingly difficult to keep up with the volume of warriors who were medevaced to Landstuhl. This ultimately hampered any real consistency in accountability, which then affected proper pay status.

By November 2005, finance battalions throughout Europe were each staffed with two to three soldiers to assist with reviewing wounded warrior pay accounts in their respective community or country. However, most of the work was done remotely, with small operations as far away as Belgium and Italy, all of which made this mission additionally challenging.

In May 2006, a US news article was published about injured warriors medically evacuated from combat zone areas owing money to the government due to the continuation of receiving combat zone entitlements.[3] Just a few weeks prior, on April 27, 2006, nine people had testified about this issue before the House Government Reform Committee. The hearing reported nearly 900 wounded soldiers owing more than $1.2 million in government debt.[3] Further reviews found that between 2002 and 2005, nearly 1,300 soldiers who were wounded and left the Army, or who were killed in action, had debts totaling $1.5 million.[3]

Because of this initial lack of a centralized tracking system, combat pay entitlements were not immediately adjusted when soldiers were medevaced from theater. Sometimes it was weeks or even months before the system caught up with this change in status. At that point, military pay entitlements were then stopped after their true effective date, and the pay system automatically calculated a debt for this time period of "overpayment" of combat pay entitlements when the soldier was no longer in combat.

The pay system also generated a Leave and Earnings Statement that reflected amounts owed to the US government as advanced debt. Warriors were receiving a letter in the mail notifying them of this debt that they now owed to the US government. Options were provided on how to repay the debt, such as:

- making one lump sum payment,
- having the debt prorated for the same amount of time the erroneous pay continued, or
- applying for a remission or cancellation of debt.[4]

Debt of this magnitude was financially devastating for soldiers and their families. The effects were far-reaching because bills could not be paid, and credit ratings were damaged. It was particularly difficult for those warriors who had sustained permanent injuries precluding them from returning to duty. Changes were put in motion to address this problem and prevent future recurrences of soldier debt.

The 266th Finance Command provided full-spectrum finance and accounting services in USAREUR. The command oversaw the numerous finance battalions sent into Kuwait, Afghanistan, and Iraq to provide financial support to joint and combined theaters, establish banking processes, and oversee contractor support for rebuilding and refurbishing these countries. Because of the 266th Finance Command's vast number of deployment missions, and the overwhelming volume of soldiers medevaced to LRMC, the DFAS Europe team assumed the wounded warrior pay mission at LRMC in July 2006. Originally hired as temporary employees to replace the military finance staff at LRMC, DFAS Europe staff also worked with minimal resources. Their office was located on the second floor of the Deployed Warrior Medical Management Center (DWMMC) trailer, complete with recycled furniture and tight office space. Warriors on crutches or in wheelchairs were instructed to ring a bell for service, which alerted a technician to come and provide assistance.

An onsite visit by the director of DFAS Europe initiated positive changes. Plans were developed for a designated office area within the hospital itself, better accommodating wounded warriors and families. The DFAS Program Manager for Wounded Warrior Pay strongly reiterated the need for a fully staffed operation in a more suitable work environment and insisted on better financial support for these soldiers. The goal was to create a team of civilians who would focus on assisting wounded warriors at LRMC.

By May 2007, the current Wounded Warrior Pay Office at LRMC was established. Renovations of a former day care center included providing easy access for soldiers in wheelchairs and adequate space to maintain customer privacy. The mission developed into a complete proactive measure across the Army. The permanent staff consisted of a supervisor with four technicians. The 266th Finance Command continued to provide military support with an officer in charge, and the noncommissioned officer in charge was staffed through the DFAS Indianapolis Mobilization Support Office.

In August 2007, the decision was made to expand the finance team's customer service office and enhance its technical knowledge and proficiency. Although the primary mission remained proper pay of combat zone entitlements, this expansion of services resulted in nearly $400,000 in back pay for various entitlements in soldiers' accounts.[5] This addition was also a source of great satisfaction and employee morale. This office eventually became a recognized model by DFAS for all wounded warrior finance teams.

In September 2007, the LRMC operations coordinated with the 266th Finance Command's Wounded Warrior Pay Office to ensure a seamless transition for those warriors departing LRMC for various locations throughout Europe. Soldiers with less severe injuries received appropriate care at LRMC and then either transferred back to their garrison communities throughout Europe for additional medical care, or returned to their deployment location. The two teams still continue to work together to provide thorough support to Europe-based wounded warriors.

In May 2008, pay and allowance continuation (PAC) was approved for up to one year from the date of injury for those soldiers assigned to Warrior Transition Units (WTUs). These units had been established by the Army at major military medical facilities around the world to provide both logistical and personnel support for those ill and injured warriors needing at least 6 months of further medical or rehabilitative care. The new PAC regulations brought significant financial changes for wounded warriors, including the following[1]:

- Pay includes incentive payments and combat zone entitlements that soldiers are receiving at the time of the WTU assignment.
- Pay is tax free for inpatient status and for the month if the warrior is admitted as an inpatient for reasons related to MEDEVAC. Tax-free status can apply for rehospitalization up to 2 years after the end of the conflict.
- Pay is taxable for outpatient status for the duration of assignment to WTU. Outpatients also receive a PAC per diem ($3.50/day) for incidental expenses paid in a travel settlement when the warrior is released from the WTU.
- Combat zone entitlements stop at the end of the month when warriors are released from the WTU.

In May 2009, DFAS Indianapolis established the Debit Card Travel Advance Program to support families using Travel and Transportation Orders issued by the Department of the Army's Casualty Affairs Office. This was another advantageous change that greatly benefited families. Orders were issued for families traveling to LRMC and returning home; or traveling to LRMC and then traveling with the soldier for further medical care to either Walter Reed National Military Medical Center in Bethesda, Maryland, or Brooke Army Medical Center in San Antonio, Texas. Orders were also issued for families if a soldier was not expected to survive, allowing them to come to LRMC and be with their dying family member. The family was also given the option of returning home directly after the death of their loved one or traveling first to Dover Air Force Base, Delaware, for the Dignified Transfer of Remains. To date, the LRMC Wounded Warrior Finance Office has provided 242 family members with debit card advances totaling more than $131,000. The process is completed within an hour and includes preparation of the final travel claim, ensuring that the family does not have to struggle with unfamiliar forms (DD 1351-2 Travel Voucher or Subvoucher). Advances are collected with the payment processing. This is upfront cash that is loaded onto the debit card for per diem expenses, such as meals and incidentals. In many cases, these advances significantly reduce financial stress at a very difficult time for families.

Shelley Ohlendorf recalls one story in particular as a poignant reason why this mission is so important. A mother of a dying warrior wanted to be with her son in his last hours. He was kept on life support in the intensive care unit (ICU) at LRMC until she arrived. With Shelley's help, travel orders were issued, and the complicated process expedited to unite this mother and son in his last moments of life. Traveling alone, and several flight delays later, she arrived to be with him. Shelley remembers the place in the ICU where this mother sat holding her dying son in her arms. As nurses removed the mechanical support keeping him alive, this mother read to her son from his favorite childhood book, *Clifford the Big Red Dog.* With the sound of a familiar soothing voice echoing a beloved memory from his past, this valiant warrior drew his last breath in the loving arms of the woman who had given him life.

IMPLEMENTATION METHODS

When any service member becomes ill or sustains injury in a hostile fire pay area, or as a result of a hostile fire act, they are medevaced to LRMC. Like many units, the work of the wounded warrior finance office begins long before the C17 arrives at Ramstein with a new group of sick and injured soldiers. The preparation process is tedious, and the attention to detail is meticulous. The team reviews each flight manifest and the supporting Patient Movement Records to obtain the social security number (SSN) of each arriving patient. Each SSN is then run through both the active duty and reserve component pay systems to verify all Army patients. This review ensures that each injured warrior is receiving the proper combat zone entitlements and family separation allowances as applicable. If discrepancies are noted, they are addressed with the warrior and, if necessary, his or her deployed unit leader is contacted to assist with proper documentation to ensure that appropriate pay adjustments are made.

The Wounded Warrior Finance Office works closely with the Mission Team at Ramstein to ensure that they meet each arriving flight to account for and brief the arriving warriors. Regardless of patient status, this is the initial finance team that wounded warriors meet. All outpatients from every branch of service are briefed upon arrival to LRMC. The finance team explains that their direct support is to the Army and that other branches have wounded warrior pay support in CONUS. It is a bit more complicated for inpatients because their medical status determines whether a finance team member is able to meet with them on the day of arrival. If initial contact cannot be made, the team makes daily attempts to meet with inpatients to provide updates and answer questions as long as they are at LRMC. In medically critical cases, family members are brought to the bedside and briefed on financial matters. The main mission is to ensure the prevention of combat zone entitlement debts, and alleviate this stress and worry for wounded warriors.

Once the finance team verifies the arrival of all Army warriors, they establish an account for each soldier in the Army-wide WIA database, and provide a status of his or her combat zone entitlements and incentive pay. This database then serves as an audit trail of the warrior's arrival and departure from LRMC. It is updated by LRMC Wounded Warrior Pay Office staff with confirmation of departure. Accounts are then transferred to the soldier's prospective Wounded Warrior Pay Office or annotated as a return to deployment location.

Assistance is also provided with transfer of funds on the Eagle Cash card, a debit card associated with service members' direct deposit accounts. This card can be used to load or unload funds from a US Treasury Department kiosk at LRMC. The finance team is available to assist with pay inquiries or review Leave and Earnings Statements because they have found that many warriors do not really understand their pay structure. Soldiers and escorts often arrive with no money or any way to access cash. The finance team provides a casual payment of up to $200 per week to enable service members to purchase necessary items and enjoy the various opportunities at LRMC and the surrounding area. The finance team keeps track of this cash advance that is later recouped from their regular paycheck.

All wounded warriors discharged from LRMC will outprocess. At that time, the finance team meets with each soldier to answer any pay-related questions, provides updates on their combat zone entitlements, and ensures continued monitoring of their pay accounts for proper payment. All wounded warriors transferring to a medical facility for continued care are informed that another Wounded Warrior Pay Office will now pick up and provide this continued support, and will assist with travel pay for deployment and MEDEVAC processes. The LRMC finance team will continue to monitor proper pay for those soldiers returning to their deployment location.

From point of arrival at LRMC, to point of designated departure, the Wounded Warrior Pay Office supports each soldier through every step of this process. The combination of professional financial support, vigilant monitoring, and premier customer service has eliminated untold financial stress for these wounded warriors and their families. This office is the quintessential example of "mission accomplished!" All team members see this unique job opportunity as a life-changing, rewarding honor serving our nation's heroes.

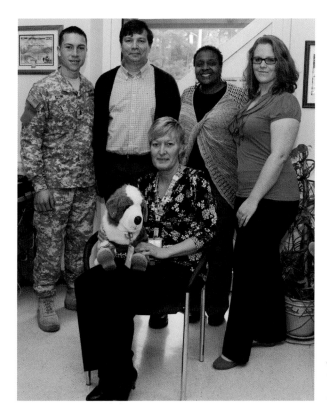

Dedicated staff of the Wounded Warrior Finance Office, Landstuhl Regional Medical Center, 2014.

Photograph courtesy of the Public Affairs Office, Landstuhl Regional Medical Center.

Leadership Staff

- *One GS 9 military pay supervisor.* Because the Wounded Warrior Finance Office does not take any holidays, the person in charge ensures that the operation is covered 365 days a year. Organization, flexibility, and multitasking with efficiency and ease are certainly important job requirements for the supervisor. What is even more essential, however, is a genuine understanding of what the wounded warrior's journey from combat to hospital bed has entailed, as well as a relentless commitment to the mission based on that understanding. This is the catalyst driving the team to provide the highest quality of service and attention. Strong communication skills are also important for this role. At any given moment, the supervisor interacts with the finance team, wounded warriors, families, personnel at LRMC, finance teams at other deployed locations, and DFAS Indianapolis. Responsibilities for this position include the following:

— hire staff;
— ensure that training is complete for both staff and wounded warriors regarding pay adjustments and transactions;
— establish the weekly schedule and on-call roster for around-the-clock coverage;
— establish strong rapport with other Landstuhl offices and other deployed finance teams to facilitate the MEDEVAC process for all warriors, and expedite problem-solving if there are complications with pay;
— help staff with travel claims and advances for families;
— liaise with DFAS to report if system problems, reports, or pay issues are interrupting the daily mission;
— prepare monthly reports; and
— brief all VIPs who visit LRMC—coordinate as needed with the 266th Financial Management Support Center (FMSC), which provides additional personnel support.

- *Four GS 5/6/7 military pay technicians.* Each technician is cross-trained on all operational processes within the office. This has created a work environment that is flexible, challenging, and growth oriented. Each team member operates with a great deal of care and compassion when providing patient briefings, which is the strength of the foundation for the team's high-quality service. Responsibilities for this position include the following:
  — prepare the pay analysis for each arriving warrior, making necessary pay adjustments based on patient status;
  — update accounts in the WIA database;
  — process the casual pay recoupments for Army customers, preventing loss of funds from these payments; and
  — assist Europe-based warriors with their travel claims if their deployment has ended.
- *Two finance soldiers from the 266th (FMSC).* The additional support from the FMSC has been mutually rewarding. FMSC has been the primary pay agent providing casual pay for wounded warriors and escorts. These two positions, usually an officer in charge and a soldier, assist with pay analysis for arriving flights, patient briefings, and in- and outprocessing of all warriors coming through the office.

Equipment and Technical Support

Equipment and technical support consist of the following:
- furniture and office supplies;

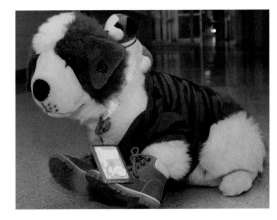

Mascot Barry, a pup in camouflage ready for a day in the trenches at the Wounded Warrior Finance Office.

Photograph courtesy of the Public Affairs Office, Landstuhl Regional Medical Center.

- wounded warrior entitlement handbooks and business cards;
- computer, duty cell phones, and safes;
- information management office support from LRMC and the 266th FMSC—the LRMC team assists with all interior computer complications, and the 266th FMSC team assists with all complications related to the finance system (often, both offices interact to ensure minimal interruption of operations since it is understood by both ends that the finance office works under time-sensitive requirements).

LESSONS LEARNED

"Look for Barry." These are the words soldiers will hear when they ask someone for the location of the Wounded Warrior Finance Office. The cheery, big-faced, St. Bernard stuffed animal is the first smile they will see when they make several rights and lefts, and finally wind down multiple hallways to find the office. It is definitely not the last. Barry is the office's official mascot and represents the friendliness, hospitality, quality service, and commitment to mission of the entire staff. The operational goal of this office is to successfully track all pay-related adjustments and alleviate financial stress. Wounded warriors need to focus on healing. The success of this office lies not only in the hard work that accomplishes this goal, but also in the hearts that are behind it.

Successes

- *Accountability.* This team has maintained 100% accountability of all Army wounded warriors arriving to and departing from LRMC, including soldiers readmitted to German hospitals. This has tremendously decreased the likelihood of combat zone entitlement debts from occurring.

- *Financial audits.* There were no combat zone-related debts that occurred in more than 40,000 accounts since 2007. Additional audits have been conducted in the months following the arrival of soldiers at LRMC to ensure that the combat zone entitlements are accurate (according to patient status).
- *Follow-up.* DFAS Indianapolis is notified of any discrepancies caused by system processes or delayed or possible erroneous action by the receiving Wounded Warrior Pay Office (many of the warriors are transferred to CONUS) to ensure that the necessary pay inputs are made. The continuation of combat zone entitlements are verified if the wounded warriors return to theater to complete their mission.
- *Communication.* To ensure accurate communication and thorough follow-up, each incoming flight to Ramstein that transports sick and injured warriors to LRMC is met by a member of the finance team to make certain that incoming patients are aware of the Wounded Warrior Pay Program. Each patient is provided with a *Wounded Warrior Pay and Entitlements Handbook* to guide them throughout their medical care. The pay status of each incoming soldier is researched by a technician prior to arrival at LRMC. Soldiers are immediately notified of any pay discrepancies. The resolution process then begins as soon as the soldier is able to complete the necessary DWMMC in-processing and come to the finance office for assistance.
- *Inpatient soldiers.* Inpatient soldiers are offered the same services with the understanding that patient acuity and medical care are the first priorities. The goal is to try to meet and brief every inpatient within 72 hours of arrival to LRMC. Patient visit logs are prepared on a daily basis to ensure that those capable of receiving a finance briefing are assisted with any pay inquiries and entitlement discrepancies. They are also reassured that their pay is not affected for the duration of inpatient status, even if transferred to CONUS for further care.
- *Morale.* The impact of these finance briefings is far-reaching. They allow many warriors to concentrate on getting better rather than focus on financial stress or concerns. Warriors are surprised and appreciative of the friendly, professional, and thorough customer service this team provides. In addition, they gain a new respect for finance operations. It is often difficult and upsetting to see the level of injuries of wounded warriors. The supervisor ensures that every team member first be informed of the medical acuity and types of injury before meeting with each inpatient warrior. This prepares them ahead of time for what to expect and has enabled the team to meet each soldier with compassion

and professionalism. It is often these simple details that make all the difference.

- *Leave and Earnings Statement.* An in-depth explanation of the Leave and Earnings Statement and current pay entitlements status is provided. Many soldiers really do not understand the entire process, nor do they have the time to ensure that they are actually being paid correctly. The finance office spends a lot of time resolving pay discrepancies, and 99% of their investigations have resulted in back pay.

- *Family assistance.* The Wounded Warrior Finance Team has played a significant role in helping families of wounded warriors. When critical situations arise, Department of the Army Casualty Operations staff expedite the passport process so that families can be at LRMC within a day. Debit card advances of more than $131,000 have been given to 242 family members. Travel entitlements for the LRMC portion of the trip are processed for families, and include a daily allowance for meals and incidentals. Prior to this assistance by the finance office, families had to pay for personal expenses up front. Although they were eventually reimbursed, this put a stressful burden on many families who simply did not have available cash to travel and be with their injured family member. This assistance has made all the difference in the world. Families are also provided with pertinent information, such as finance briefing, medical status, and programs that are specific for various types of injuries. The office also provides cash payments to wounded warriors and escorts from all branches of the service. Normally, these are cash advances of $200 per week maximum and are later processed for collection from the next paycheck. To date, the finance office has issued $725,000 with no loss of government funds because of strict internal controls and thorough review of overall office procedures.

Challenges

- *Staff and budget constraints.* Variations in flight arrivals and an ever-changing OPTEMPO (operational tempo) require a 24/7/365 operation. There is a 24-hour on-call technician and an office duty roster covering weekends and holidays to ensure that all medevaced soldiers are met upon arrival at LRMC. Budget constraints now restrict the availability of finance technicians to meet flights arriving after 1600 hours on weekdays or at any time on Sundays, if there are less than five Army outpatients. To ensure that these patients are provided with the same excellent customer service, a list of outpatients is sent to the Medical Transient Detachment staff to send the soldiers to the office the next business day.

Welcome to Germany

Anticipation mounts as the CASF (Contingency Aeromedical Staging Facility) team waiting at Ramstein Air Base watches the C-17 loom closer. Things move quickly and efficiently from the moment the wheels touch the ground, and the mammoth slate gray plane comes to a stop. Like the jaws of a shark, the rear of the C-17 opens wide and deep. At first glance, onlookers can only visualize massive amounts of cargo that a group of soldiers are unfastening and moving out for transport back to Landstuhl Regional Medical Center (LRMC). Walking up the ramp of the plane and behind the cargo, the scene tells another story, one that is actually quite astonishing. For the 10-, 12-, or 17-hour flight that it took to fly to Germany from Afghanistan, the C-17 was a fully equipped flying hospital, complete with an airborne intensive care unit.

The eyes take in what the mind is trying to quickly process. Nurses and doctors are hovering around stretchers where wounded warriors lie, some attached to ventilators, oxygen, monitors, and tubing of every sort and life-sustaining purpose. Limbs and heads are swathed in bandages, and sometimes it is hard to even see the person amidst all of this intervention. The walls of the C-17 are gigantic outlets for the electrical support needed for intricate machinery, generators for back-up support, and computers to track necessary information. It is clear that a complex and organized system is in place to quickly and safely transport these seriously injured patients from the hospital in the air to the hospital on land.

At the same time, an array of camouflage is moving about on the plane, soldiers glad to be stretching their legs and walking after so many hours sitting and strapped into a jump seat. They are also patients, primarily ambulatory, needing medical care at LRMC for a variety of reasons. Some of the soldiers are non-medical escorts coming from their downrange units to accompany a particular individual. What they all generally share in common is that they are tired, hungry, and glad to have landed.

The CASF team that waited with anticipation quickly moves into action, each person knowing their designated role. Seriously injured patients are the first priority to be transferred off the C-17 and onto the blue-converted ambulance bus (AMBUS). All seats have been removed to make room for as many gurneys as possible, secured into place with straps stretching from ceiling to floor. Patients continue to be monitored by the Critical Care Air Transport Team (CCATT) that escorted them from downrange on the C-17. The driver is given the thumbs-up to proceed, and the AMBUS then begins its 20-minute trek from Ramstein to LRMC along bumpy, curvy roads.

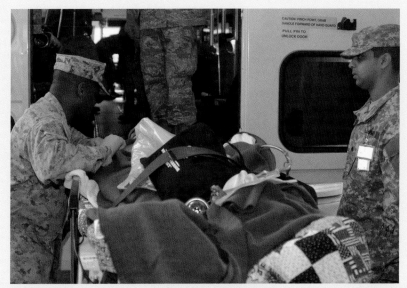

Chaplain Ronald Pettigrew (*left*) welcomes a patient as he is being transferred from the ambulance bus to Landstuhl Regional Medical Center.

Photograph courtesy of the Public Affairs Office, Landstuhl Regional Medical Center.

Simultaneously, another team has also been preparing for the C-17 arrival. At 0600 hours, the sun is still resting at LRMC, and the morning frost on the grass glistens in the light shining from the awning outside the emergency room doors. Shoe style and camouflage color reveal that every branch of the military is represented in this group: Army, Navy, Air Force, and Marines. Some carry clipboards with notes they review, while others cradle a warm cup to help offset their shivers from the cold morning air. They are a combination of medical staff, liaisons (or Liaison Noncommissioned Officers), administrative staff, volunteers, and chaplains. They also have their designated role once the wounded warriors arrive. Neither time of day nor rain, snow, or sleet ever interfere with what has become a daily routine in a decade of war.

The AMBUS pulls in front and stops, the back doors swing open, and an immediate protocol of movement begins. Lines are formed on either side of the doors, four staff to a side, arranged from the tallest to the shortest. Great care, respect, and precision are in evidence as each stretcher is gently passed from the AMBUS, down the line to each person, and onto a wheeled gurney. Instructions can be heard, such as "move left," "be careful of the IV [intravenous line]," or "got it!"

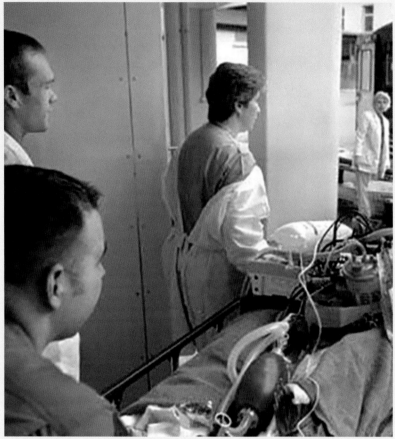

Army Captain Karla Clarke, an Intensive Care Unit nurse at Landstuhl Regional Medical Center, assists in transporting her patient to a bus for air transport. August 2007.

Photograph courtesy of Soldiers' Angels Germany.

When the stretcher is secured to the gurney on the ground, the chaplain is the first to greet each wounded warrior. Some patients are conscious, whereas others are not. The chaplain reaches for a hand, or even just a finger, amid the dizzying array of tubing, machinery, and bandages. Regardless of their level of awareness, religious denomination, or military rank, each wounded warrior hears the words, *"Welcome to Landstuhl [first name of soldier], you are safe."* A short prayer is then offered. In those few seconds, a human connection is made, and the whisper of a comforting voice reminds them of home.

Inpatients are incorporated into the daily visit log preparation for the team to conduct bedside briefings. This then requires additional follow-up to ensure that all needs are met.

- *Communication delay.* When discrepancies are identified, all efforts are made to resolve them with the soldier within 2 days. In most cases, this is possible. If warriors arrive with no combat zone entitlements on their pay accounts, verification of deployment date from the soldier's unit is needed. There are many soldiers who do not have contact information with them, so extensive measures are undertaken to obtain a good point of contact to assist with the necessary confirmation of deployment date. Unfortunately, not all units are able to respond to the request for assistance. When no documentation is received to resolve the discrepancy, combat zone entitlements are started and are effective from the day soldiers are medevaced. Back pay is processed for the soldier. A note of explanation about the issue is made in the WIA database to ensure that all back pay is processed with the assistance of the forwarding Wounded Warrior Pay Office. Each wounded warrior has an account that transfers to each assigned location.

- *Europe Warrior Transition Unit assignment process.* When soldiers are transferred to CONUS for continuous care, they report to a WTU. Determination is later made to release soldiers to their units or keep them in the WTU while their care continues. For Europe-based soldiers, the process is in reverse; they *first* return to their units and *then* must apply for WTU status. Approval of these applications averages 3 to 5 months. This affects the PAC entitlement, often causing PAC entitlement inquiries to then be made through Human Resources Command (HRC). This office is responsible for the Army's management of assignments and personnel. The HRC is the determining authority on PAC issues. For those warriors not receiving PAC, all inquiries are made through the HRC in conjunction with the DFAS Indianapolis Wounded Warrior Pay Management Office. If full PAC status is approved for these warriors, back pay of entitlements is processed. But this presents an accountability and pay issue for warriors in Europe that can take months to resolve. There is no current solution other than the PAC inquiry process, but a suggestion to have the WTU assignment process reevaluated for Europe-based soldiers is being considered.

Because this mission has so many moving parts in caring for wounded warriors, there are often destination diversions in CONUS of which LRMC is not informed. A soldier may be set for transfer to a certain facility, but health complications can arise that result in the transfer of that soldier to another location. The Wounded Warrior Finance Office has access to the manifest listing names of all service members transferred from LRMC to the next medical facility. This manifest, however, is not updated once they leave LRMC. Eventually, the LRMC finance office is contacted by a CONUS Wounded Warrior Pay Office because amended travel orders are required if diversion occurred from the original orders issued. This delays the travel settlement process for these warriors. Thus, upon request from the CONUS Wounded Warrior Pay Office, a request for amended orders is sent to the LRMC Movement and Orders Team. The affected soldiers are paid as soon as the amendments are issued. The location of warriors is what drives their entitlements. Accuracy is therefore imperative. If these destination diversions occur with little or delayed follow-up by the accepting medical facility, Wounded Warrior Pay Office entitlements can be affected.

Sometimes soldiers are given bad news regarding their health and whether they will ever be able to return to duty. Some have suffered terribly from their injuries. Sometimes soldiers are simply worn down from the reality of war. Every member of the finance team is only too happy to serve as an interim family member or friend to warriors far away from their unit and from their own families. A candy dish on every desk, sweets from the local bakery or a staff member's oven, an endless supply of hugs, and always, sincere words of thanks and encouragement; this is the atmosphere that soldiers walk into after "meeting" Barry at the door. The LRMC Wounded Warrior Finance Team deeply believes that wounded warriors and their families deserve the best support possible. They pride themselves on delivering the whole package: financial support, professional expertise, and attention to every necessary detail, all wrapped in the human essence of kindness and compassion. Staff is not afraid of long hours and hard work—whatever it takes to serve our warriors who have served our country. This is the mindset instilled in this team. The Wounded Warrior Pay Office is an integral part of the Landstuhl story. Since its development in 2006, countless soldiers and their families have benefited from this mission and the outstanding people who have carried it through.

For the most up-to-date content, visit the Wounded Warrior Finance Office website at www.dfas.mil/militarymembers/woundedwarrior/woundedwarriorpay.html.

ACKNOWLEDGMENT
We wish to thank Shelley Ohlendorf for her assistance with this chapter.

REFERENCES
1.   Wounded Warrior Pay Management Team, Defense Finance and Accounting Service. *Wounded Warrior Pay and Entitlements Handbook*, January 2013.
2.   Christensen J, Hanrahan M, Burghardt S. One can only imagine: easing the burden of financial strain on Wounded Warriors and their families is a commitment that DFAS personnel take most seriously. *Armed Forces Comptroller.* Fall 2010; Vol 55, No 4.
3.   Government Accountability Office. *Military Pay: Military Debts Present Significant Hardships for Hundreds of Sick and Injured GWOT Soldiers.* Washington, DC: GAO; April 27, 2006. GAO report number GAO-06-657T. http://www.gao.gov/assets/120/113657.html. Accessed December 15, 2014.
4.   Department of the Army. *Remission or Cancellation of Indebtedness.* Washington, DC: DA; April 29, 2009. Army Regulation 600-4.
5.   Wounded Warrior Finance Office. Monthly reports. Landstuhl Regional Medical Center, Germany,

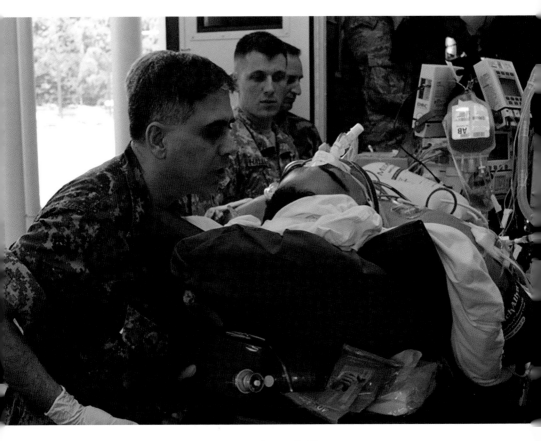

Trauma patient from "downrange" arriving from Ramstein Air
Base via "AMBUS" (ambulance bus).

Photograph courtesy of the US Army.

CHAPTER SEVEN

Trauma

*World-class health care routinely envisions what could be . . . so that the
extraordinary becomes ordinary and the exceptional routine.*

— KENNETH K. WIZER, MD, MPH

---

*The early trauma program encompassed all surgical disciplines,
including general surgery, orthopedics, and the other surgical subspecialties,
as well as the medicine subspecialties of pulmonology, critical care, infectious
disease, and gastroenterology. The goal of the trauma program was to
establish timely multidisciplinary care. This was initially accomplished
informally without an explicit organizational structure. There was no
organized performance improvement or patient safety program specific to the
care of the trauma patient, despite the exponentially increasing numbers of
severely wounded casualties arriving at Landstuhl Regional Medical Center.*

Throughout the history of modern warfare, the military medical response
has had to continuously adapt to both the increasing lethality of weapons
used and geographic constraints. Despite these challenges, the military
has mobilized robust medical assets to austere and hostile locations throughout the
world.[1] As a result, combat casualty care has significantly improved, and mortality
rates are historically lower.

The development of sophisticated critical care air transport capability has
further enhanced patient outcomes through the transcontinental evacuation of
critically ill patients out of combat theaters to hospitals within the United States
at unprecedented speed. To manage large numbers of severely injured patients
across three continents, a sophisticated trauma system spanning multiple roles of
care had to be developed. Understanding how Landstuhl Regional Medical Center
(LRMC) developed as a key military medical treatment facility (MTF) within this
global continuum of casualty evacuation is an integral lesson learned for future
facilities.

BACKGROUND
Development of the Trauma Program at Landstuhl
Regional Medical Center

The trauma program at LRMC was developed to provide optimal care for combat casualties. Prior to the wars in Iraq and Afghanistan, LRMC rarely cared for traumatically injured patients. Clinicians with varying levels of experience provided care in their own independent manner, and communication between the different roles of care was nonexistent. The events of September 11, 2001, and then combat operations in Afghanistan and Iraq brought about an abrupt need for change. These events subsequently led to the development of the world's largest and most complex inclusive trauma system, stretching over thousands of miles and three continents.

As the largest US military healthcare facility in Europe, LRMC found itself in a unique position as the common link between US Central Command (CENTCOM), whose areas of responsibility included Iraq and Afghanistan, and the continental US (CONUS) medical facilities. Although the primary source of casualties came from CENTCOM, LRMC was also strategically located as an evacuation facility for the US Africa Command (AFRICOM) and the US European Command (EUCOM). The intent of Landstuhl's trauma program was to streamline the process of care between the turbulence of deployed facilities to the safe haven of an MTF in Germany. LRMC also served as the evacuation hospital for CONUS medical centers.

The early trauma program encompassed all surgical disciplines, including general surgery, orthopedics, and the other surgical subspecialties, as well as the medicine subspecialties of pulmonology, critical care, infectious disease, and gastroenterology. The goal of the trauma program was to establish timely multidisciplinary care. This was initially accomplished informally without an explicit organizational structure. There was no organized performance improvement (PI) or patient safety program specific to the care of the trauma patient, despite the exponentially increasing numbers of severely wounded casualties arriving at LRMC. Although some measures of PI and patient safety were accomplished through the surgical and professional diligence of individual providers, the overall lack of structure, organization, and objective standards resulted in inconsistent practices and variable outcomes.

It was therefore determined that the trauma program required the expertise of an experienced trauma program manager (a nurse), as well as the leadership of a fellowship-trained surgeon in critical care who could successfully develop and implement the goals of the trauma program. Implementation of evidence-based trauma practice, strong management, recruitment of experienced trauma staff, and

Catchment area for Landstuhl Regional Medical Center. This area includes CENTCOM, AFRICOM, and EUCOM—three of the nine combatant commands.

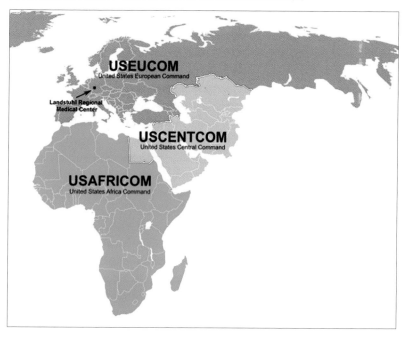

establishment of a model trauma plan aligned with the criteria set by the American College of Surgeons (ACS) eventually led to the verification of LRMC as an ACS Role 2 trauma center in 2007. This received full support from the LRMC command and approval of the Europe Regional Medical Command. The mission and vision of the LRMC trauma program were to decrease patient morbidity and mortality, which mirrored the mission and vision statements of LRMC:

> *To provide world class comprehensive and compassionate care to our Nation's injured Warriors and families, through a maintained and ready healthcare force that seeks, thrives on, and embraces change while accomplishing the mission.*[2]

Optimum patient care could only be accomplished through a multidisciplinary team approach using the collaborative efforts of all services. Civilian leadership and military nurse leadership were particularly instrumental in providing and maintaining this continuity of care because of the severe nature of combat injuries, the immediacy of care required, and the high physician turnover related to deployments and short reservist rotations.

American College of Surgeons Committee on Trauma Verification Process at Landstuhl Regional Medical Center

The ACS trauma verification program at LRMC was established through collaboration with military and civilian trauma system experts using the ACS Committee on Trauma (COT) manual, *Resources for Optimal Care of the Injured Patient, 2006.* This manual outlined more than 240 criteria for optimal resources needed to provide consistent and contemporary trauma care, and served as a guide for the ACS COT trauma center verification process by outlining trauma center requirements.[3] Trauma care in general crosses multiple medical disciplines. Trauma care within the military structure also had to cross interservice barriers between the Navy, Army, and Air Force to provide care and transportation of trauma patients across three continents.

Early in the conflicts in Afghanistan and Iraq, military services did not have an integrated trauma system. Each service had its own version of predeployment training and trauma experience. There was also a lack of effective communication between roles of care. Each service had a different emphasis on trauma, as evidenced by a disproportionate number of trauma and critical care-trained surgeons and nurses. In addition, not all services had a dedicated trauma consultant under their respective surgeons general. Furthermore, there were no senior nursing positions dedicated to trauma program systems.

In addition, there was a general lack of institutional knowledge regarding trauma programs and trauma systems organization. Therefore, hiring an experienced civilian trauma program manager was vital to the success of LRMC achieving ACS verification. The trauma program manager hired at LRMC had a master's degree in nursing and decades of experience in the clinical and management aspects of major civilian trauma centers, as well as extensive experience in the ACS verification process. This individual also provided the necessary expertise to perform systematic and comprehensive gaps and barriers analyses, and could implement appropriate changes and interventions as assessed.

In addition, a number of senior civilian trauma surgeons played a significant role in supporting the growth of LRMC as a trauma center.[4] The Senior Visiting Surgeon Program, co-sponsored by the American Association for the Surgery of Trauma and the ACS COT, provided the ability for recognized senior civilian leaders in trauma and surgical critical care to visit LRMC. This program also provided for an active interaction and flow of information between the civilian and military communities. More than 60 senior visiting surgeons volunteered time and expertise in caring for the wounded and in mentoring military surgeons and staff.

When it was verified as a Role 2 center in 2007, LRMC became the first medical facility outside of the United States to be verified by the ACS as a trauma center. The hospital was reverified in 2010. Both research and graduate medical education were enhanced, and LRMC achieved verification as a Level I trauma center in 2011 with multiple accolades and no deficiencies.

Implementation of the Trauma Program—Part I: Trauma Program Organization

The Department of Trauma and Critical Care was composed of the Trauma Critical Care Service and trauma program staff. The Trauma Critical Care Service had up to five trauma critical care surgeons and three critical care medical physicians. The trauma program staff included two trauma registrars, five trauma PI staff members, four research coordinators, and three support staff.

Trauma programs include the following components:

- combat casualty care,
- a trauma registry,
- PI and patient safety safeguards,
- education,
- injury prevention efforts,
- rehabilitation,
- research, and
- graduate medical education.

Three of these components are described in detail below because they specifically apply to the military and LRMC.

COMBAT CASUALTY CARE

Management of casualties coming directly from the combat theater required a special diligence and specific understanding of combat trauma because the injuries encountered differed in both mechanism and severity compared with those seen in civilian trauma centers. Causes of such injuries included the following:

- improvised explosive devices (IEDs) encountered on foot patrol with blast injury (combined primary blast injury, thermal injury, blunt trauma from being thrown, and penetrating fragment wounds),
- gunshot wounds sustained on roofs or hilltops with subsequent falls and concomitant blunt trauma,
- gunshot wounds sustained by vehicle drivers traveling at high speeds followed by collision or rollover, and
- IED blasts encountered in armored vehicles with subsequent rollover into canals resulting in near drowning.

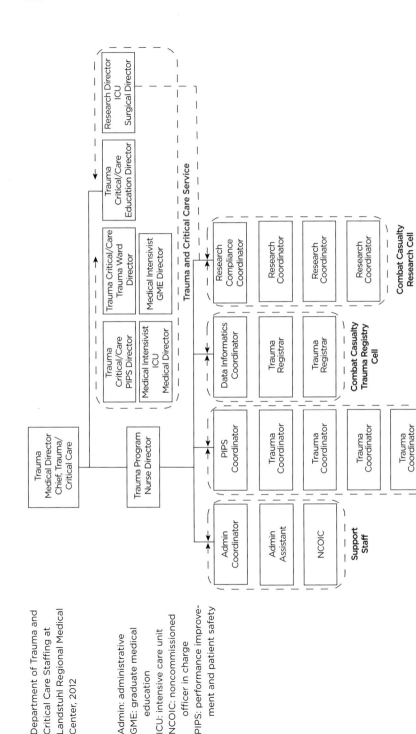

Department of Trauma and Critical Care Staffing at Landstuhl Regional Medical Center, 2012

Admin: administrative
GME: graduate medical education
ICU: intensive care unit
NCOIC: noncommissioned officer in charge
PIPS: performance improvement and patient safety

The mechanisms and weaponry used during the conflicts in Iraq and Afghanistan also changed over time. For example, IED blasts in vehicles were a significant injury mechanism seen in casualties during Operation Iraqi Freedom (OIF) from 2003 to 2009. Vehicles utilized early in this theater were less heavily armored, resulting in frequent penetrating wounds and burns. Later in the conflict, the vehicles became more heavily armored. In response, the IEDs then became more powerful. This resulted in the creation of a blunt injury pattern with calcaneal fractures, pelvic fractures, vertebral fractures, and traumatic brain injuries resulting from vehicles being violently thrown into the air and then landing.[5]

When the drawdown in OIF occurred, there was a shift and the majority of casualties began coming from the Afghanistan theater. Because of terrain challenges and changes in military tactics in Afghanistan, foot patrols became more common. More IEDs were encountered on foot than had been seen in OIF, and the effects of primary, secondary, and tertiary blast effects became commonplace, resulting in spinal cord injuries and multiple limb amputations with severe penetrating perineal and pelvic injuries. An increase in the incidence of invasive fungal infections was also seen at the same time.[6] The severity and multisystem nature of these injuries presented constant challenges to military physicians. These continuously changing patterns of injury and their resulting complications required a comprehensive PI process to develop and maintain best practice guidelines and standard operating procedures (SOPs).

As in any military installation, there was a frequent turnover of provider staff at LRMC. This situation created an ongoing need to reteach best treatment practices with each incoming medical team. The development of clinical practice guidelines and SOPs improved patient outcomes and minimized variations in practice. The trauma program was responsible for monitoring provider adherence and compliance with best clinical practice guidelines and SOPs. Deviations from these practices had to be documented and investigated immediately. This ensured greater consistency in practice and improved clinical outcomes compared to earlier in the conflict.

TRAUMA REGISTRY

Initially, there was no method to adequately capture and utilize trauma data to improve outcomes and develop lessons learned. In an effort to improve care throughout the trauma care continuum, the Joint Theater Trauma System (JTTS) was developed under the Center for Army Strategic Studies and Army Institute of Surgical Research. The JTTS then implemented the Joint Theater Trauma Registry (JTTR), which was approved by the Army surgeon general in 2002. Initially, collection of combat casualty data was independently completed via spreadsheets or homegrown databases at multiple military MTFs in theater, as well as in CONUS. Over time, the JTTR matured into a single, web-based data entry system that could be accessed from military MTFs in theater, as well as at LRMC and CONUS facilities. The trauma registry was used to code and sort information for analysis and reports through the use of either system/process checks (audit filters), or review of universally defined morbidities (eg, pneumonia or infections), in order to drive evidence-based PI and quality assurance. This registry resulted in a standardized data collection system for all roles of combat casualty care and allowed for well-defined data elements, automatic calculation of the number and percentage of those with specific diagnoses, categorization and scoring of injury severity, and the use of standardized coding procedures.

PERFORMANCE IMPROVEMENT AND PATIENT SAFETY SAFEGUARDS

The trauma PI and patient safety processes required the continuous gathering of data. Any part of the trauma care system at LRMC that did not perform well was identified through a network of communications that included trauma service morning reports, intensive care unit (ICU) and ward rounds, self-reporting, concurrent chart reviews, and trended registry reports.

Assessment of the PI process transcended several continents and actually began prior to the patient's arrival at LRMC. Acute resuscitation and damage control procedures were initiated and frequently completed in theater. Patient care then continued across Europe and back to facilities in the United States. Communication across continents with different time zones further exacerbated the challenge of this widespread geographic distribution of patient care delivery. Once the patient left LRMC, PI issues were also identified in CONUS. The creation of a forum for communication across the continuum of care was vital to the PI process.

In 2005, the LRMC trauma program initiated a unique PI process through the worldwide Trauma Clinical Video Teleconference (VTC). The VTC was held on a weekly basis, and included video and audio participation from the point of injury to the CONUS facilities. It also included leaders of the Tactical Combat Casualty Care system and members of the JTTS. During this teleconference, issues of communication, operative and critical care, transport and equipment, PI, and opportunities to enhance care were presented openly. All members of the LRMC trauma team participated in the VTC, and the PI issues identified were forwarded to the LRMC trauma program director, the JTTS medical director, or the trauma medical directors in CONUS.

POSITION DESCRIPTIONS
- Trauma Medical Director
  The specific duties and responsibilities of the trauma medical director are outlined in detail in the ACS's *Resources for Optimal Care of the Injured*

Patient, 2006.[3] Specific to the military, the trauma medical director was an active duty trauma critical care surgeon who also served as the chief of the Department of Trauma and Critical Care. The general responsibilities included establishing the operational management of the day-to-day clinical care of trauma patients. The overarching goal was to support the integration of the LRMC trauma program across the JTTS, while simultaneously maintaining trauma center standards established by ACS. Leadership duties and responsibilities of the trauma medical director also included development of the strategic vision for trauma operations at LRMC, as well as integration of the trauma program across the continuum of care.

Participation in PI and peer review activities coordinated between LRMC and the JTTS and CONUS trauma programs was essential. LRMC was in a unique position to identify trends in outcomes and process changes from within theater. LRMC provided the necessary continuity in reporting these trends because the trauma surgeons changed every 3 to 6 months in theater, and every 3 years at LRMC. From this vantage point, the LRMC trauma director was able to identify and communicate variations from clinical practice guidelines, SOPs, or unanticipated complications present on arrival. LRMC has benefited from the efforts of several trauma medical directors over the 11 years of combat operations.

- Trauma Program Nurse Director (Trauma Program Manager)
  The specific duties and responsibilities of the trauma program manager (TPM) are outlined in detail in the ACS's *Resources for Optimal Care of the Injured Patient, 2006.*[3] Specific to LRMC, the trauma program nurse director (TPM equivalent) was a civilian employee and a registered nurse. An extensive background in trauma program management at a civilian ACS or state-verified Role 1 or 2 trauma center was a prerequisite for this position. Interestingly, the Department of Defense (DoD) did not have a trauma program nurse director or other trauma program position available to active duty nurses.

  This position required strong communication skills because the trauma program nurse director collaborated with the trauma medical director while also interfacing with LRMC military leadership, medical staff, nursing staff, and the regulatory agency of the ACS Committee on Trauma Verification.[3]

  The TPM was responsible for strategic trauma center planning, supervision of the operational budget, management of all departmental nonprovider staff, leadership of the ACS verification preparation process, and the educational and skill development of the professional staff in matters related to trauma care. Both the trauma program director and the trauma program nurse director interfaced with key departmental directors, and were representatives of the trauma program to hospital leadership. The TPM also had the essential role of integrating with JTTS program managers in other unified commands, primarily CENTCOM and NORTHCOM (US Northern Command). As the trauma program matured, the manager's responsibilities extended throughout EUCOM and, in conjunction with the director, the TPM developed the EUCOM component of the worldwide JTTS.

Implementation of the Trauma Program—Part II:
Characteristics of the Patient Population and
Flow of Patient Care

The military trauma system was visualized as one hospital across three continents. After point-of-injury care occurred in the combat theater, patients had the majority of their acute injuries stabilized at Role 2 or Role 3 military MTFs. A typical Army Role 2 MFT was composed primarily of a forward surgical team that could resuscitate and surgically stabilize patients for transfer to the next level of care. Army Role 3 MTFs were stationary hospitals located at major airfield hubs in the combat zone with enhanced capabilities, such as computerized tomography (CT) scanning, angiography, magnetic resonance imaging (MRI), and a multitude of specialty surgeons. As soon as they were stabilized for transportation, patients were transferred to a Role 3 staging facility. Throughout combat operations during OIF and Operation Enduring Freedom (OEF), key in-theater facilities at Balad, Iraq, and Bagram, Afghanistan, prepared patients for transfer from the combat hospital to Landstuhl.

Patient flow differed at LRMC compared to a traditional trauma center within the United States, where injured patients typically arrive from the point of injury and are taken directly to the emergency department (ED). Once the LRMC trauma team received notification of incoming patients, the on-call trauma surgeon triaged the patients pre-arrival based on the patients' movement medical records (a short synopsis of the patient's injuries and care) received from the Role 3 MTF. This information enabled patients to be transported directly from the aircraft to the appropriate location within the hospital. A trauma activation was initiated for any patient who became unstable or met certain neurological or hemodynamic instability criteria. This alerted LRMC medical staff to prepare appropriate, high-level resources to best care for that patient. Medically unstable patients were transported directly to the ICU. Patients not undergoing activation

Timeline of transport and roles of care after combat injury—*Role 1*: field care. *Role 2*: limited in-theater resuscitative capabilities. *Role 3*: highest level of in-theater care, includes many surgical and medical specialties. *Role 4*: hospital near area of operations, but outside theater.

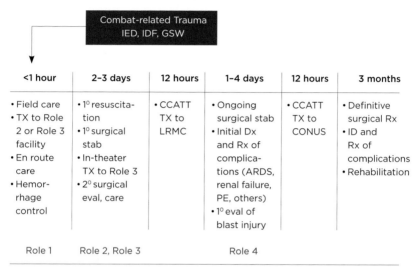

| | Combat-related Trauma IED, IDF, GSW | | | | | |

<1 hour	2–3 days	12 hours	1–4 days	12 hours	3 months
• Field care • TX to Role 2 or Role 3 facility • En route care • Hemorrhage control	• 1° resuscitation • 1° surgical stab • In-theater TX to Role 3 • 2° surgical eval, care	• CCATT TX to LRMC	• Ongoing surgical stab • Initial Dx and Rx of complications (ARDS, renal failure, PE, others) • 1° eval of blast injury	• CCATT TX to CONUS	• Definitive surgical Rx • ID and Rx of complications • Rehabilitation
Role 1	Role 2, Role 3		Role 4		

ARDS: acute respiratory distress syndrome
CCATT: Critical Care Air Transport Team
CONUS: continental United States
Dx: diagnosis
eval: evaluation
GSW: gunshot wound
ID: identification

IDF: indirect fire
IED: improvised explosive device
PE: pulmonary embolism
Rx: treatment
stab: stabilization
TX: transport

were admitted either directly to the ICU or to the general medical/surgical in-patient unit based on the clinical information relayed. Patients admitted to the ICU usually required ongoing resuscitation and further operative procedures. This intermediate stop at LRMC after a 6- to 10-hour transport mission from the combat theater was both mandatory and clinically essential because many critical patients could not tolerate the long flight directly from the combat theater back to the United States (at least 16 hours).

LANDSTUHL REGIONAL MEDICAL CENTER
TRAUMA PATIENT POPULATION

Although the majority of trauma patients cared for at LRMC arrived by air transport from Iraq or Afghanistan, patients were also occasionally injured on the base at Landstuhl (Army) or Ramstein (Air Force). These patients were transported to LRMC by the Ramstein Air Base ambulance service. Occasionally, patients transported themselves to the ED, and sometimes locally stationed injured service members were transported directly to the LRMC ED by German civilian ambulance crews. All injured patients were evaluated in the LRMC ED for hemodynamic stability (a tiered trauma response), and a trauma activation was called, if appropriate. Patients who required admission were admitted to a surgical service or had a trauma consultation.

More commonly, aeromedical transportation of trauma patients from OIF or OEF (3,000 miles) or to CONUS (4,000 miles) was provided by a combination of aeromedical evacuation (AE) and Critical Care Air Transport Teams (CCATTs). The CCATT operated as an ICU in the cabin of a fixed-wing aircraft during flight, adding critical care capability to the US Air Force AE system that did not exist in the first Gulf War (see Chapter 8, Nursing, for a detailed discussion of the history and utilization of CCATTs).[7]

The typical patient transported by the CCATT had undergone initial evaluation and operative management in one or two hospitals in the combat zone. These patients were often still in their early postresuscitative stage after injury at the time of their transport to Germany. Less severely injured patients who did not require critical care en route were transported by AE teams. These teams were composed of nurses and technicians with specialized training in AE. All in-flight patient concerns were immediately relayed to LRMC. The AE and CCATT teams had activation criteria for both trauma and critical incidents. Part of the halo effect of being a trauma center was that 50% of the activations that did occur were not for trauma patients, yet these patients benefited from this well-organized system. This enabled a more robust medical response immediately on arrival of the patient into the ICU.

Aeromedical transportation of patients in the local German area was provided by civilian assets. The German Red Cross (Deutsches Rotes Kreuz or DRK) also provided rotary wing transportation of trauma patients in the local area. If patients required critical care during these transportations, the DRK platforms (helicopter or ambulance) could be staffed by local critical care physicians. Of note, LRMC did not serve as a base station for local emergency medical services operations.

Implementation of the Trauma Program—Part III:
Trauma Service—Clinical Care

The structure was in place for the trauma service to care for injured patients as soon as they arrived at LRMC. Multiple disciplines were involved, including general surgery, orthopedics, neurosurgery, emergency medicine, critical care, pulmonology, infectious diseases, radiology, and surgical subspecialties.

Patients with multisystem injuries were admitted to either the ward or the ICU, but were always under the direct management of a general or trauma surgeon. Patients who suffered single-system injuries were admitted to the appropriate specialty service with mandatory consultation to the trauma service for certain indications. All trauma patients, regardless of location in the hospital or the admitting service, were monitored and tracked by trauma coordinators.

In the ICU, assessments were performed on all patients by the ICU team, composed of one trauma surgeon, one general surgeon, one intensivist (medicine or pulmonary critical care), rotating residents (from US-based military residencies, typically two on service most months), and a physician assistant or acute care nurse provider. The ICU team leader was a trauma surgeon, and the individual daily assessment and plans were communicated to the ICU team leader during morning rounds.

The trauma ward service was composed of a single attending general or trauma surgeon and two physician assistants. All aspects of the patient's care were managed by the attending surgeon. Each morning, the trauma service made rounds on the ward, and ICU physicians, trauma nurse coordinators, physician assistants, perioperative nurse director, ICU nurse director, case managers, and chief of surgery attended as well. All systems issues and complications in the trauma service were discussed to capture significant PI events.

The trauma medical director oversaw all aspects of multidisciplinary care provided to trauma patients at LRMC through several parallel channels. The trauma service morning report and reports by the trauma coordinators were key forums for day-to-day operations. The trauma coordinators acted as the functional eyes and ears of the trauma medical director by visiting patient care areas daily, observing care plans, and identifying key issues that needed the attention of the trauma medical director. Trauma coordinators had access to the trauma medical director at any time to convey concerns.

Other channels of information to enhance management and patient care included the trauma morbidity and mortality conference, the weekly patient feedback VTC (encompassing providers from Iraq/Afghanistan to CONUS), and multidisciplinary peer review conferences.

SUBSPECIALTY SURGEONS

Because of the significant specialization and increasing sophistication of catheter-based therapeutics, a fellowship-trained vascular surgeon was required at LRMC to provide optimal care to patients suffering from vascular injury. At the beginning of operations in Iraq, vascular surgery care at LRMC was provided by rotating reservists. This was not sustainable because of the small numbers of vascular cases at LRMC. Beginning in 2007, members of the Society for Vascular Surgery (SVS) volunteered to provide needed expertise during 2-week rotations at LRMC in which they were credentialed to supply services as civilian Red Cross volunteers. Since that time, more than 80 SVS members have rotated through LRMC, serving as consultants in this increasingly specialized area.

Neurosurgery was another vital specialty required for all trauma centers. At LRMC, neurosurgical services had been provided through a variety of means. During the initial phase of the conflict (2001–2004), neurosurgical patients were transferred to a local German facility for their care. Patients who required acute neurosurgical services arrived at Ramstein Air Base and were transported directly to either the German military hospital in Koblenz (200 km) or the civilian trauma center in Homburg (22 km). Neurosurgeons at both of those facilities also had privileges at LRMC and could attend to patients onsite (although this occurred rarely). Beginning in 2004, members of the American Association of Neurological Surgeons offered their services as Red Cross volunteers and provided much of the needed care to injured patients. Starting in 2006, neurosurgeons from the Navy and Army Reserves provided continuous, 24-hour-a-day care in conjunction with a contracted civilian neurosurgeon. Availability and standardization of neurosurgical trauma care have been the greatest challenges of the trauma program.

INTENSIVE CARE UNIT

The trauma ICU system is based on a closed model, wherein the patient was admitted to the trauma service that directed the patient's care.[8] Patients who underwent resuscitation and surgical stabilization in theater arrived daily, and were admitted directly from the flight line to the ICU. Multidisciplinary rounds were conducted daily with multiple specialists, including infectious disease, pulmonary/ critical care, pharmacy, respiratory therapy, nutrition, and trauma coordinators. A critically important role of the trauma service was to determine when the patient was stable enough to be evacuated to a Role 4 MTF in CONUS, such as Walter Reed National Military Medical Center in Bethesda, Maryland, or San Antonio Military Medical Center in Texas. This decision was challenging because the physician had to balance the benefits of being in a definitive care setting close to home in the United States, while also considering the potential dangers of an 8- to 10-hour transcontinental flight. However, as the trauma program and trauma services at LRMC evolved, almost all the necessary ICU supportive care was available, making it possible to hold patients until they were stable for transport by CCATT to CONUS. Most patients spent 2 to 3 days hospitalized at LRMC. Despite changes in the two conflicts in the Middle East, both ICU and hospital admissions to the trauma service remained relatively stable with approximately 40 ICU admissions per month, though there was a steady rise in the Injury Severity Score.

Trauma admissions to the intensive care unit by month correlated with the Injury Severity Score from January 2007 through June 2012

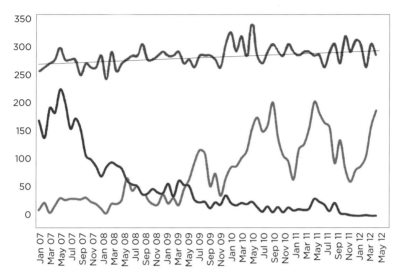

blue line: Operation Enduring Freedom
red line: Operation Iraqi Freedom/Operation New Dawn
green line: average intensive care unit Injury Severity Score
thin black line: linear (average intensive care unit Injury Severity Score)

Medical Records

Maintaining accurate and timely medical records from downrange through CONUS was essential for the continuity of care. During the early phases of OIF and OEF, medical records were kept on paper charts that followed the patient through multiple roles of care. These records were sometimes scant, unintelligible, or frequently misplaced during the chaos of intertheater transport. During busy combat periods, many surgeons wrote the operative procedures performed on the patient directly onto the patient's dressings with permanent markers. Communication regarding the condition of incoming patients was challenging, so LRMC staff developed and implemented the Joint Patient Tracking Application (JPTA). This was a secure, military, web-based application that allowed providers from combat theaters to communicate critical information regarding resuscitation and operative interventions. It also allowed the upload of operative notes, photographs, discharge summaries, and supporting documentation in theater, at LRMC, and in CONUS. JPTA was touted by the providers as an excellent and user-friendly method to maintain a consecutive record and move critical information

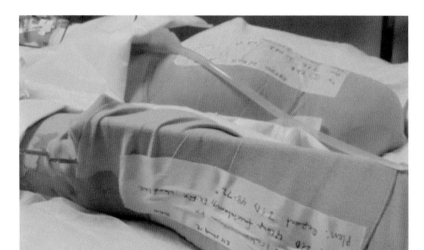

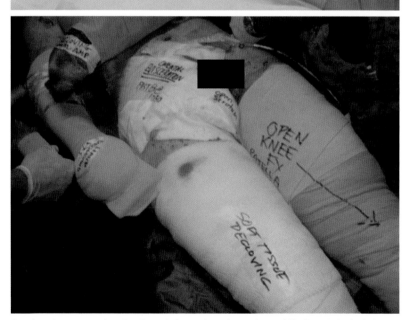

Combat documentation. Pertinent information about site and findings is included on dressing to facilitate communication between roles of care.

through the various roles of care. JPTA was reliable, allowed for quick transfer of information between sites, and was modifiable to meet the changing needs of the combat theater.

The JPTA system morphed into a vital tool used by all roles of care. With great effort, that system was then integrated with Medical Communications for Combat Casualty Care (MC4) in 2009 and became the Theater Medical Data Store (TMDS). TMDS was a secure, web-based patient tracking and management tool used to collect, manage, analyze, and report data on patients arriving at all MTFs from their deployed locations. It provided administrators and medical personnel with the ability to view the current status of patients as they moved through all roles of care. Providers used the TMDS to transmit key medical information to the next caregivers along the continuum. This improved the medical staff's ability to anticipate and plan for the needs of incoming patients, as opposed to waiting until they arrived.

The original JPTA program was developed at LRMC for a minimal cost, but the current TMDS is now operated and managed by DoD. All hard copies of intra-theater and LRMC paper medical records (including downrange documentation) and follow-up information were scanned to a HIPAA (Health Insurance Portability and Accountability Act)-compliant, web-based site at LRMC to facilitate the collection of data into the trauma registry, support research efforts, and develop improved methods of care. Laboratory and radiology results were also included.

Radiology

At the beginning of the wars, there were no diagnostic images forwarded from the combat theater, and official radiology reports were scant. Out of necessity, most injured patients arriving from downrange were reimaged. Eventually CT scan images were loaded onto compact discs that were sent along with the patient's hard-copy medical records. In 2006, a digital radiology system called PACS (Picture Archiving and Communication System) was installed to store and retrieve images, and an interface between the combat theaters and LRMC was established. This required a manual "push" of the films over the Internet to LRMC, as well as a manual "pull" from LRMC. Radiology technologists came into the hospital at night to have films available by the time the wounded warriors arrived the next day. However, sagittal and coronal reconstructions could not be transferred because of large bandwidth requirements; thus, the LRMC radiologist completed the reconstructions on studies performed in theater. The culmination of efficient and reliable data transmission significantly decreased the need to perform repeat radiological studies or procedures between roles of care.

LESSONS LEARNED

During times of military conflict, experiences gained by military physicians have contributed to the advancement of civilian trauma care. There has been a significant effort to promote dissemination of lessons learned from pivotal clinical experiences over the last decade at LRMC. Over the last few years, more than 50 peer-reviewed publications related to patient care at LRMC have been published in the medical literature. Many of the successes of the trauma program at LRMC were born from the challenges encountered in the earlier years of conflict and the interventions that were created to address them.

End-of-Life Care

In 2004, DoD issued a directive that all military personnel receive organ donation-related information and that the names of those personnel interested in participating be documented. The directive also stated that all military hospitals should affiliate with a local organ procurement organization for education and procurement purposes. LRMC developed an affiliation with the Deutsche Stiftung Organtransplantation (DSO), the national organ procurement organization in Germany. Standards for determining brain death and patient donor eligibility according to the DSO mirrored DoD policy. In addition, the DSO did not participate in donation after cardiac death, which is acceptable practice in the United States. Patients were declared brain dead at LRMC in accordance with local policy.

Families were often present during the brain death determination at LRMC. This rapid response occurred with the assistance of the service member's deployed unit, who notified the family in cases of catastrophic injuries, and also with the assistance of the Departments of the Army, Navy, and Air Force, which expedited the issuance of passports, if necessary. Once the family was reunited, confirmation was documented regarding the patient's preference for organ donation. The family was approached by a trained physician or registered nurse who was not participating in the care of the patient. These individuals underwent 4 hours of training conducted by the DSO on how to approach families for organ donation. Once the patient's organ donation status was confirmed, the German organ procurement team conducted the organ harvest at LRMC, with vigilant attendance of an Armed Forces Medical Examiner. Between 2001 and 2010, there were 93 combat casualty deaths at LRMC primarily from severe head injuries. The organ donation conversion rate for that period of time was 85% for those who were eligible for donation, with 105 organs recovered.[9] As a comparison, the US Organ Procurement and Transplantation Network reported a national conversion rate of 73% for 2012.[10]

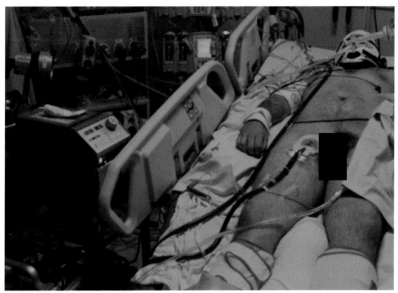

Veno-venous extracorporeal membrane oxygenation at Landstuhl Regional Medical Center.

Acute Lung Rescue Team

The Acute Lung Rescue Team (ALRT) was the only team in the DoD with the capability to transport combat casualties with severe lung injury.[11] The development of acute lung injury and acute respiratory distress syndrome significantly complicated evacuation of critically ill and injured casualties. In the past, patients with acute lung injury remained in theater until either their condition improved or they died. The ALRT, which was housed at LRMC, performed missions to transport seriously ill patients from the EUCOM, CENTCOM, and AFRICOM theaters of operations. Members of the team included both surgical and medical intensivists, ICU nurses, and respiratory therapists, all trained in CCATT. Additional therapeutic options available to the ALRT included advanced modes of ventilator support using specialized transport ventilators (eg, volumetric diffusive respirator percussive ventilation), inhaled prostacyclin, and extracorporeal membrane oxygenation (ECMO) capability.

The ALRT transported patients more critically ill than those transported via CCATT. Patients transported by ALRT had a predicted mortality of more than 70% and an average oxygen need of 93% FiO_2 (fraction of inspired oxygen), compared with a CCATT patient who typically had a predicted mortality of 35% and an average oxygen need of 53% FiO_2. The ALRT was activated for both trauma (60%) and nontrauma diagnoses (40%). Trauma-related diagnoses

Number of activations of the Acute Lung Rescue Team from 2005 to 2012
Cx: cancelled (if cancelled because patient died, death occurred prior to arrival of
the team)

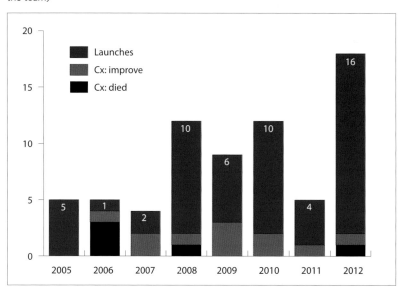

Pulmonary support used by the Acute Lung Rescue Team

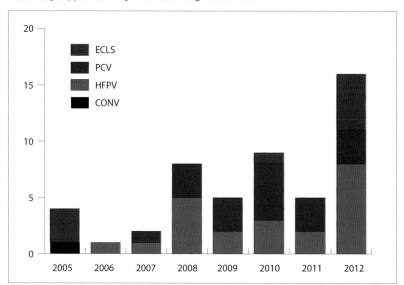

CONV: conventional ventilation   HFPV: high-frequency percussive ventilation
ECLS: extracorporeal life support   PCV: pressure control ventilation

included blunt pulmonary contusion, blast and thermal inhalation injuries, near drowning, and penetrating chest injuries. Nontrauma patients with diagnoses of eosinophilic pneumonitis, sepsis, pneumonia, multiple organ failure, and postcardiac arrest were also transported.[11,12] Between 2005 and 2012, the team was activated more than 60 times.

Extracorporeal Membrane Oxygenation

ECMO was an infrequently needed, but potentially life-saving, mode of support for patients with severe pulmonary failure.[11,12] Patients suffering from lung injury due to combat were potentially excellent candidates for ECMO because most were young and sustained a form of lung injury (blast injury) that was typically reversible over a relatively short period of time. In concert with colleagues from the University Hospital Regensburg, the ALRT initiated ECMO multiple times between 2005 and 2012. After evaluation by members of the ALRT, patients who met eligibility criteria for ECMO were typically cannulated by the ALRT surgical intensivist at Role 3 facilities in theater (or at other medical facilities in EUCOM or AFRICOM). After cannulation and stabilization, patients were then transported to LRMC. Once stabilized at LRMC, patients were transferred to the University Hospital Regensburg for respiratory care until they could be weaned off ECMO. The survival rates were excellent, with 100% of patients surviving until ECMO was removed and 85% of patients surviving 30 days from that point.

Deep Vein Thrombus Screening and Prophylaxis

A systemic prevention program for deep vein thrombus (DVT) was one of the first JTTS clinical practice guidelines enacted because of a perceived high DVT/ pulmonary embolism rate. In conjunction with the JTTS director's in-theater program, LRMC began an aggressive DVT prevention protocol that included early chemical prophylaxis, sequential compression stocking use, and DVT screening on all ICU patients and other high-risk groups. In a PI analysis (postinitiation of the DVT screening program), the rate of DVT was 14.1% (80 patients with DVT), and the rate of pulmonary embolism was 4.42% (25 patients with pulmonary embolism). The newly identified rates of thromboembolic events were significantly higher than those identified prior to this aggressive screening program.[9] Further analysis identified that femoral venous catheters, in common use at this time, were a significant risk factor for the development of DVT. Efforts were then enacted to remove them as early as possible. Furthermore, all patients with DVT and pulmonary embolism were treated with therapeutic anticoagulation or inferior vena cava filters if contraindications to anticoagulation existed.

Invasive Fungal Infections After Combat Injury

Infections had been a problem in the combat injured since the beginning of the conflicts. An increase in invasive fungal infections in the immune competent service member has been noted.[13] These infections included the unusual pathogens (unusual for the immunocompetent host) *Mucor* and *Aspergillus*. The occurrence of these infections in patients after injury was associated with significant morbidity. The clinical picture of progressive ongoing tissue necrosis in the wounds of a critically injured patient who demonstrated signs of systemic inflammatory response was a common presenting scenario. An aggressive approach of early diagnosis and initiation of appropriate local and systemic therapies to treat infection improved outcomes. A number of risk factors were identified for invasive fungal infections in the combat injured, including dismounted (patrolling on foot rather than in a vehicle) blast injury, above-the-knee traumatic amputations, extensive perineal/pelvic injury with the need for massive transfusion, and injury location in the Afghanistan Sangin River Valley.

Recognition of this problem at LRMC led to the development of a blast injury protocol that was initiated in those patients at particular risk for an invasive fungal infection. This protocol included histological evaluation and microbiological culture of tissue during the first debridement after arrival from theater. Histological evaluation included fungal staining and evaluation for plant material and foreign material in debrided tissue. This early histological evaluation significantly facilitated identifying patients with fungal infection.

Incomplete Fasciotomy

Because of the increased incidence of missed and incomplete fasciotomies, a retrospective review of 336 combat casualties undergoing 643 fasciotomies in Iraq, Afghanistan, and LRMC was performed. Patients requiring a fasciotomy revision at LRMC had a fourfold increase in mortality. Additionally, patients had increased rates of amputation (31% vs 15%) when they required a fasciotomy revision. The most commonly unopened compartments were the anterior and deep compartments of the lower leg.[14]

This led to an ALARACT (or All Army Activities) specifying that Role 2 and 3 military MTFs should liberally perform complete fasciotomies when indicated.[15] Prophylactic fasciotomies should be performed prior to transport for at-risk extremities. Delaying transport for 24-hour observation was recommended for those casualties at high risk for developing compartment syndrome and in cases where the surgeon decided against immediate fasciotomy. This also led to significant changes in emergency war surgery courses and other predeployment training programs that now emphasized the two-incision, four-compartment release method of relieving the lower leg compartments.[15] Thus, there was a major decrease in overall missed compartment syndromes and adequate compartment releases.

Revision of Brooke Army Medical Center
Burn Resuscitation Algorithm

Complications such as overresuscitation and abdominal compartment syndrome were seen in seriously burned patients transported through the various roles of care. Identification of this problem led to a multidisciplinary development of a resuscitation algorithm and Burn Flow Sheet. The algorithm was later modified by the US Army Institute of Surgical Research ICU team. This was promulgated throughout the system with the publication of a burn resuscitation clinical practice guideline by the JTTS. Weekly utilization of the algorithm and flow sheet, with appropriate feedback to deployed providers at Role 2 and 3 facilities at the theater-wide VTC, led to a significant reduction of complications from overresuscitation.[16,17]

THE FUTURE: MAINTAINING TRAUMA CENTER VIABILITY AND CAPABILITY

Returning to prewar conditions raises major concern both for Landstuhl and, by implication, other DoD facilities that may serve as Role 4 hospitals. Our wounded warriors deserve world-class care. Such excellence in care was a significant challenge for Landstuhl at the beginning of the current conflicts. It required nearly 6 years to establish a mature trauma program and trauma system at LRMC. In retrospect, it would be faster and more efficient to expand an *existing* trauma program that remained in continuous readiness to handle a large influx of severely injured patients during outbreaks in hostilities within the combatant commands. This type of approach would also provide the agility to support shorter conflicts (the expected norm) without the need to expand over the years of the conflict. Such an approach allows many of the processes and services that would already be engaged in a trauma system—such as operating room readiness, critical care service, the massive transfusion protocol, PI, and the trauma registry—to immediately expand because many of those processes would already be in place. Building on the lessons learned at LRMC, the institutional knowledge and process of trauma care, as well as the engagement of necessary services (eg, blood bank and neurosurgery), would be present and active in this situation.

How would such a facility, operating at a lower level, be kept active? The area serviced by Landstuhl includes Africa, Europe, and the Middle East. It is certain that there will continue to be low-level conflicts in these areas that will contribute to the need for trauma services and a trauma system, such as the attack on the American diplomatic compound in Benghazi, Libya, on September 11, 2012. In addition, there are significant numbers of service members and dependents within the catchment area. A significant portion of beneficiaries injured in EUCOM could be sent to LRMC once their acute injuries were stabilized. It is likely that this level of activity would support activities at Landstuhl commensurate with an ACS Role 3 trauma facility and support involvement of the multidisciplinary medical and ancillary care critical to its function. This approach should also be applicable to other regions of the globe where the US military has a presence. These opportunities would serve to maintain a Role 4 military MTF viability as a trauma center. To achieve that goal, the trauma program staffing should be incorporated into the Table of Distribution and Allowances (TDA) of all Role 4 military MTFs. Many of the roles of the trauma program staff could be accomplished by active duty military personnel. To maintain the manpower necessary to provide trauma center and trauma systems expertise, each branch of military service will need to make this type of professional development a priority.

There are two technology/capability fixes that would aid in the functioning of a Role 4 facility during times of lower operational tempo. The *first capability* is telemedicine, which is increasingly being used for patient care in rural areas and for complex conditions. Telemedicine has significant potential benefit in the military setting, especially in the areas of critical and subspecialty care. The department of surgery at LRMC has pioneered a novel telemedicine clinic in otolaryngology with remote clinics in Germany. The specialty providers are able to perform, via video, examinations of the ear, nose, and mouth performed by a surrogate provider (primary care physician or nurse practitioner). There is also a plan to test this technology in the combat theater with burn patients. The ability to project specialty expertise to austere locations could help fill gaps during mobilization to contingency operations. Similarly, ICUs at LRMC can be equipped with monitors to provide remote intensive care consultation and monitoring. This practice has been shown in studies to reduce mortality, reduce ICU lengths of stay, and increase adherence to best care practices.[18]

The *second capability* is aeromedical transport. There is currently significant capability to transport critically ill patients through the CCATT program. This program allows evacuation of patients across long distances to the Role 4 facility. The high volume of patient transfer (more than 8,000 patient movements) and associated low morbidity are testaments to a finely tuned training program. Therefore, the CCATT concept must continue to be used because it will become an asset for peacetime initiatives. The advanced experience of the LRMC-based ALRT serves as both a model for the DoD and the civilian sector.

The input and efforts of multiple groups have significantly improved the current US military trauma system compared to previous conflicts. If remaining challenges were addressed and improved upon, care for injured service members would be significantly improved in the future. These challenges include the following:

- *Electronic health record.* Communication between roles of care has significantly improved. However, the military medical system, like many health systems, struggles with integrating multiple electronic record systems to provide a longitudinal medical record across the entire continuum of care. This is a significant challenge to overcome across continents. The consolidation of one unified record, which includes all radiological images, is critical to improving communication and care.
- *Performance improvement.* The DoD JTTS has made significant strides in PI efforts across the continuum of care. However, there continues to be difficulty in identifying and tracking complications across the system. An example of this is the patient who develops a pulmonary embolus at a Role 4 facility in CONUS after receiving suboptimal anticoagulation at another Role 4 facility prior to arrival. Current tracking mechanisms do not allow for routine reporting of this type of complication back to LRMC, which then hinders subsequent PI efforts up and down the care continuum.
- *Trauma program.* Further definition of the role and importance of the trauma program within the military hierarchy and across the various military services would significantly facilitate function. The DoD readiness organizations have always emphasized individual unit training and equipment, but have been very slow to recognize the importance of trauma systems and trauma programs. This was evidenced by the need to hire civilian personnel to manage the trauma program at LRMC. Training and maintaining active duty nurses in the skills necessary to manage a trauma program and a trauma PI program within the institution would provide continuity and bridge gaps within the military system.
- *Turnover rate.* Turnover continues to limit the development of institutional memory at most military facilities. The estimated annual turnover at LRMC is 40%.[9] A cap of only 25% turnover of personnel (to include reservists) every 6 months should be implemented in order to maintain optimal clinical performance and growth.

ONE HOSPITAL ACROSS THREE CONTINENTS

LRMC is in a unique and vital position as the Role 4 facility providing combat casualty care to all patients injured during combat operations in the current conflicts. Over time, LRMC has matured into a robust and active trauma center and is perhaps the most critical example of the global care model for US combat casualty care. Nearly 100% of surviving patients injured in two theaters of operation (Iraq and Afghanistan) have passed through LRMC for additional care. The pace of modern warfare and the increasing lethality of weapons used will require the Role 4 military MTFs of the future to respond quickly and efficiently. To capitalize on lessons learned, facilities such as LRMC should maintain trauma center viability in perpetuity.

ACKNOWLEDGMENTS
Greg Beilman, MD, COL, US Army Reserve, Trauma/Critical Care Surgeon; John Oh, MD, LTC, US Army, Surgeon and Director, Trauma Program; Kathleen Martin, RN, MSN, Nurse Director, Trauma Program; David Zonies, MD, Lt Col, US Air Force, Surgeon and Director, Trauma Program; Ray Fang, MD, Lt Col, US Air Force, Trauma/Critical Care Surgeon and Director, C-STARS; Donald D. Trunkey, MD, FACS, Trauma Surgeon; Warren Dorlac, MD, COL, US Air Force, Medical Director, Trauma/Critical Care Unit and Director, C-STARS.

REFERENCES
1. Hetz SP. Introduction to military medicine: a brief overview. *Surg Clin North Am.* 2006;86:675–688.
2. Trauma program mission statement as provided by Oh J, Martin K, Beilman, G, Zonies D, Fang R, Trunkey D, Dorlac W. Landstuhl Regional Medical Center, January 2013.
3. American College of Surgeons Committee on Trauma. *Resources for Optimal Care of the Injured Patient, 2006.* Chicago, IL: COT-ACS; 2007.
4. Martin MJ, Dubose JJ, Rodriguez C, et al. "One front and one battle" : civilian processional medical support of military surgeons. *J Am Coll Surg.* 2012;215:432–437.
5. Possley DR, Blair JA, Freedman BA, et al. Skeletal Trauma Research Consortium (STReC). The effect of vehicle protection on spine injuries in military conflict. *Spine J.* 2012;12:843–848.
6. Warkentien T, Rodriguez C, Lloyd B, et al. Invasive mild infections following combat-related injuries. *Clin Infect Dis.* 2012;55:1441–1449.
7. Cannon JW, Zonies DH, Benfield RJ, et al. Advanced en-route critical care during combat operations. *Bull Am Coll Surg.* 2011;96(5):21–29.
8. Fang R, Pruitt VM, Dorlac GR, et al. Critical care at Landstuhl Regional Medical Center. *Crit Care Med.* 2008;36(7 suppl):S383–S387.
9. Statistics provided by Oh J, Martin K, Beilman, G, Zonies D, Fang R, Trunkey D, Dorlac W. Landstuhl Regional Medical Center, January 2013.

10. US Department of Health & Human Services, Health Resources and Services Administration. *OPTN/SRTR 2012 Annual Data Report: Deceased Organ Donation.* Washington, DC: HHS; 2012. http://srtr.transplant.hrsa.gov/annual_reports/2012/pdf/07_dod_13.pdf. Accessed August 2, 2015.

11. Fang R, Allan PF, Womble SG, et al. Closing the "care in the air" capability gap for severe lung injury: the Landstuhl Acute Lung Rescue Team and extracorporeal lung support. *J Trauma.* 2011;71(1 suppl):S91–S97.

12. Dorlac GR, Fang R, Pruitt VM, et al. Air transport of patients with severe lung injury: development and utilization of the Acute Lung Rescue Team. *J Trauma.* 2009;66(4 suppl):S164–S171.

13. Paolino KM, Henry JA, Hospenthal DR, et al. Invasive fungal infections following combat-related injury. *Mil Med.* 2012;177:681–685.

14. Ritenour AE, Dorlac WC, Fang R, et al. Complications after fasciotomy revision and delayed compartment release in combat patients. *J Trauma.* 2008;64(2 suppl):S153–S161.

15. US Department of the Army. *Management of OIF/OEF Casualties Requiring Extremity Fasciotomy.* Washington, DC: HQDA; May 2007. ALARACT Memorandum 106/2007.

16. Chung KK, Wolf SE, Cancio LC, et al. Resuscitation of severely burned military casualties: fluid begets more fluid. *J Trauma.* 2009;67:231–237.

17. Ennis JL, Chung KK, Renz EM, et al. Joint Theater Trauma System implementation of burn resuscitation guidelines improves outcomes in severely burned military casualties. *J Trauma.* 2008;64(2 suppl):S146–S151.

18. Lilly CM, Cody S, Zhao H, et al. Hospital mortality, length of stay, and preventable complications among critically ill patients before and after tele-ICU reengineering of critical care processes. *JAMA.* 2011;305:2175–2183.

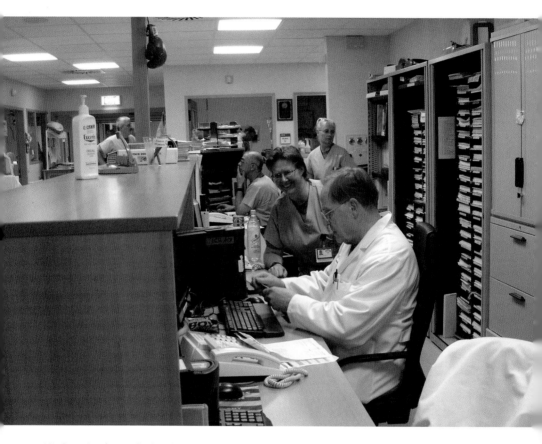

Work station for medical staff at Landstuhl Regional
Medical Center.

Photograph courtesy of CDR Kevin Kumlien, Navy reservist,
Intensive Care Unit nurse.

CHAPTER EIGHT

Nursing

Heroes are never perfect, but they're brave, they're authentic, they're courageous, determined, discreet, and they've got grit.

WADE DAVIS, PhD
ANTHROPOLOGIST AND ETHNOBOTANIST
UNIVERSITY OF BRITISH COLUMBIA

I ntensive care units (ICUs) in civilian hospitals are stressful environments. Patients are in critical condition, the workload is demanding, and noise is constant from beeping machines, monitors, and ongoing conversation between various caregivers on the clinical team. Flexibility is mandatory because a seemingly stable moment can change in an instant. A phone call from the emergency room usually means there is a new admission, maybe more than one. This brings a heightened level of activity as bed status is reviewed, changes made, and assignments added to a nurse's already stressful patient load.

Medical-surgical (med/surg) floors at civilian hospitals are also notoriously busy. Although patients are not as seriously ill as in an ICU, the volume of patients in those units can be triple. Depending on the shift, nurses can care for anywhere between five and ten patients at a time, many postoperative, and most with complex comorbidities.

Across the ocean in Germany, nurses at an American-based military hospital experience stress, critical patients, change, the need for flexibility, and tragedy at a level far beyond what is seen in any civilian hospital. After the onset of Operation Enduring Freedom (OEF) and Operation Iraqi Freedom (OIF), Landstuhl Regional Medical Center (LRMC) was transformed from a quiet, "sleepy" community hospital caring for routine medical problems to a Level I trauma center caring for thousands of combat casualties evacuated from war zones. Every administrative and clinical unit within this facility underwent rapid evaluation and change to meet the enormous and complex needs of wounded

Remembering Landstuhl

Without a doubt, the hardest part of being a nurse at Landstuhl Regional Medical Center was the emotional piece. I had worked in the neurotrauma intensive care unit at a large civilian hospital before I was deployed, and thought I was "42 and bulletproof." But this was something altogether different; these were young kids, so many of them, and with so many devastating injuries. Their lives would never be the same again, and you just wondered how they could survive all of this. It was crisis after crisis in that intensive care unit, and you were so busy that you did not have time to wrap your brain around all of the devastation, or rationalize any of it.

One story I will never forget happened early in my deployment. My patient was a young lady evacuated from Afghanistan, the only survivor in her unit after an explosion where both of her legs were blown off. In a morphine haze, she was unaware of her surroundings, and I repeated to her that she was safe in Germany. As the accident was recalled in her mind, she asked about the others in her unit, name by name. I had to deliver the news that they had died. She repeatedly asked, "Why did I make it?"I remember standing next to her bed and telling her, "I don't know why you are here, but I believe you will have the rest of your life to figure that out." It was a statement I repeated many times to other soldiers in similar circumstances who asked the same question. I don't know what made me say this to that patient, but I could only hope that she and others like her found a sense of peace and the realization that there was still purpose in their lives.

CDR KEVIN KUMLIEN, NAVY RESERVIST
INTENSIVE CARE UNIT NURSE

soldiers. Nursing responsibilities changed drastically as well. While improvements in Kevlar (DuPont, Wilmington, DE) body armor protected soldiers better than in earlier conflicts, current weaponry brought devastating injuries. Casualties rarely arrived at LRMC with just a single injury. Polytrauma, such as traumatic brain injury (TBI), multilimb amputations, blindness, burns, and penetrating wounds produced a cascading series of needs that required an intricate level of care. Four major kinds of nurses played integral roles in the lifesaving efforts of caring for wounded warriors: ICU and med/surg clinical nurses and inpatient and outpatient nurse case managers (NCMs).

BACKGROUND

Demographics became quite different for LRMC with the onset of the global war on terrorism (GWOT). Prior to 2001, the hospital primarily provided primary and tertiary care to military personnel and their families in the European

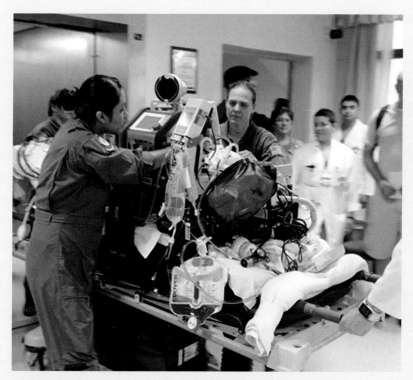

A team of nurses and doctors from Landstuhl Regional Medical Center.
Photograph courtesy of US Air Force.

theater. Hospital staffing was a combination of Army (50%), Air Force (15%), and civilian (35%) personnel.[1] The nursing department at LRMC was under the direction of the Army command. Caring for wounded warriors was certainly not a new phenomenon for military nurses. As far back as 1943, Army nurses were trained in air evacuation procedures, caring for patients from secret missions in North Africa, New Guinea, and India. The concept of transporting wounded soldiers by helicopter ambulances to frontline mobile surgical hospitals began during the Korean War, and nurses helped transport more than 17,000 of those soldiers. The helicopter system was further refined during the Vietnam War.[2]

The nurses at LRMC rose to the occasion in this military conflict. The wars in Iraq and Afghanistan, however, were straining the medical center, which remained committed to its primary purpose of treating US service members and families, in addition to caring for the deluge of injured soldiers evacuated from downrange. The workload at LRMC was most intense when the fighting was

The ten heaviest casualty months at Landstuhl Regional Medical Center: Operation Enduring Freedom/Operation Iraqi Freedom/Operation New Dawn inpatients, January 2003 to July 2013.

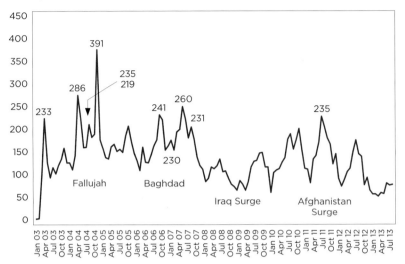

most intense. During the first attack on Fallujah, in April 2004, there were more than 400 war-related inpatient admissions, and this increased to more than 500 with the second Fallujah attack in November.[3] On average, casualties from the war accounted for 60% of the hospital census.[4] The constant flow of soldiers with devastating injuries was taking a toll on caregivers, and additional support was needed.

A plan was initiated to acquire resources from all military branches and augment the clinical staff at LRMC. This plan also freed up Army personnel, who could now be sent forward to combat hospitals where additional medical support was also needed. In October 2006, a group of 350 Navy reservists from the Great Lakes region were deployed and arrived at LRMC. This was now a true triservice initiative. There were some initial adjustments for both sides as the existing staff at Landstuhl saw the high clinical skill level of incoming reservists (corpsmen, nurses, etc) and reorganized to utilize these capabilities most efficiently. New staff had to learn various computer systems, paper charting, and the rules of the Army command. Although the challenges were great, the plan was quite successful as this dedicated, skilled, and hard-working group significantly contributed to the excellent quality of care given to wounded warriors at LRMC. The first group of Navy reservists completed their tour in November 2007 and was succeeded by another equally large reservist group who continued providing necessary medical support to LRMC. As the intensity of the war diminished, the numbers of deployed Navy reservists decreased. In 2014, the last group of Navy reservists was deployed to LRMC.

IMPLEMENTATION: HOSPITAL CLINICAL NURSING
Preparing for Arrival

> *Morning report in the ICU and the med/surg floors is suddenly interrupted by each unit clerk's voice on the intercom announcing "wheels down." There is immediate reaction to these words, a palpable change in the room demeanor as faces turn solemn, bodies tense, and heart rates increase. These two seemingly simple words impart great impact: an incoming flight from downrange has just arrived at Ramstein Air Base with wounded warriors from combat and other patients with various illnesses. They will soon be transported to LRMC. The initial silence is quickly broken by a rush of adrenaline, and the realization of all that needs to be done in preparation for this arrival.[5]*

Althugh wounded warriors arrived at any time of the day or night, this was a typical scenario for nurses who prepared for each new group of patients evacuated from theater to LRMC. During different points in the war, they heard the words "wheels down" more than once a day. Nursing teams are usually able to review the patient medical records (PMRs) 1 to 6 hours before the flight arrives at Ramstein. These records contain the patient's history, diagnosis, event of the injury/illness, and any treatment that has been given from time of injury to time of evacuation from the combat support hospital.[5] The PMR also documents the medical condition of the patient during flight, medications given, and medical equipment used. This is vital information that helps the medical team at LRMC determine which patients will be assigned to the ICU and the med/surg floor. Nurses try to anticipate what equipment they will need: additional wound care supplies and devices, patient-controlled anesthesia pumps, ventilators, chest tubes, and intravenous pumps. No pause button can be hit, no downtime can be found. There is constant movement, conversation, planning, and decision-making in anticipation of patient arrival and all that it entails. In the midst of all of this, nurses are still caring for their other critically ill ICU patients.

All trauma patients and nontrauma patients requiring mechanical ventilation, invasive monitoring, or vasoactive medications are admitted to the ICU. Beds must be made available and patient assignments shifted to accommodate new arrivals. It is not unusual for the ICU to admit six new patients from one flight, while also preparing a group of three to five critically ill patients for transport to the continental United States (CONUS) by the Critical Care Air Transport Team (CCATT).[5]

Nurses on the med/surg floors react in a similar manner upon hearing the news. They know how hectic and stressful the day is going to get. Each of the three med/surg floors may receive five or six sick and injured patients per flight.[5] These nurses are also reviewing PMRs, finding beds for new patients, obtaining proper equipment, and balancing nursing assignments. Nurses became used to making initial assessments about patient needs from the PMRs, planning how to address these needs, and then implementing and re-evaluating the assessments when they could see and touch the wounded soldier or civilian in front of them.

Arrival of Patients at Ramstein and Transport to Landstuhl

There is heightened activity at Ramstein Air Base as another group is also preparing for this arrival of wounded soldiers. Members of the Contingency Aeromedical Staging Facility (CASF) teams are there to assist with patient transport from the aircraft to the ambulance bus (AMBUS) to LRMC. CASF personnel strategically position themselves at the rear of the plane, and wait for it to open to move things along as quickly and as seamlessly as possible. First priority is given to assisting the CCATT with transferring critical patients to one AMBUS, and then less critical patients are assisted to another. During the flight, the CCATT—consisting of a critical care nurse, physician, and respiratory technician—members have cared for the complex and seriously ill patients. CCATT's role is to stay with these patients until they are received by the ICU team at LRMC. Each patient is carefully lifted onto a litter by the CASF team and taken to the AMBUS, which has been constructed to accommodate patient litters and a variety of medical equipment. Once on board, each litter is secured to a Special Medical Emergency Evacuation Device (SMEED), which is a metal platform created to hold and stabilize medical equipment, such as intravenous pumps, oxygen tanks, ventilators, suction canisters, and cardiac monitors. Before the AMBUS driver starts the vehicle, there is a round of assessments to prepare patients for the bumpy, 20-minute trip to LRMC. The CCATT nurse or doctor may bolus narcotics to lessen pain or sedate a patient to reduce intracranial pressure or decrease anxiety. It is not uncommon for monitors to alarm en route, and each situation is addressed accordingly.[5] Although this is the last stage of the journey, the AMBUS moves slowly because bumpy ground transportation is uncomfortable and difficult for patients. Finally, after multiple transports from combat field to combat hospital to a C-17, in which patients travel thousands of miles, the AMBUS makes one last turn onto "cardiac hill," the aptly named steep, forested driveway that runs straight up to the hospital from Landstuhl village. After passing through the gates, the familiar blue bus with the Red Cross sign pulls in front of the emergency department at LRMC, where another group anxiously waits to welcome the wounded warriors.

Arrival of Patients at Landstuhl

An overhead page delivers a message directing all available or designated nursing staff to the emergency department. ICU nurses and respiratory therapists wear yellow isolation gowns and protective gloves and stand ready to receive new critically ill patients. Other hospital nursing staff and NCMs are there to welcome soldiers and assist in directing them to the appropriate pre-assigned unit. The LRMC team hoists each litter from the AMBUS onto a gurney. The chaplain then welcomes all soldiers by name, whether they are awake and alert or in a coma. Critically ill patients are taken to the ICU, where CCATT members give an updated report for each patient they monitored during the flight to the respective LRMC ICU nurse now caring for those patients. Hospital equipment replaces that used on the plane, and the nurses remove the SMEED.[5]

The LRMC critical care team of nurse, physician, and respiratory therapist do their own initial assessment, and baseline laboratory tests are sent off. Critically ill patients are often unstable, in varying stages of sepsis, respiratory failure, and multi-organ failure.[5] Multitasking is essential, as orders are coming quickly and urgently from various medical disciplines. At any given moment, portable chest x-rays are being done on all intubated patients, changes are made to ventilator settings, a computerized tomography (CT) scan is needed for a patient with increased intracranial pressure, vasopressor dosages are adjusted, antibiotics are added, patients are prepped for surgery, dialysis is initiated, and fluid resuscitation is intensified.[5] Experienced nurses guide novice nurses and those who are new to the unit. All records and reports from combat facilities need to be retrieved and organized to ensure continuity of care because most patients are stabilized at LRMC and transported to CONUS within 24 to 72 hours of arrival. Those patients who are medically unstable to withstand the long air travel remain at LRMC until they are able to do so.[5]

The situation is also hectic on the med/surg units, where staff are settling patients in their rooms and retriaging them. Every effort is made to keep wounded warriors together for support and camaraderie. Sometimes a patient's medical status has altered during the flight and changes need to be made from the pre-assigned unit. At any time, the med/surg charge nurse may need to accept additional patients originally sent to the ICU who are now medically stable, or send patients who are now medically unstable to the ICU from the floor.

The med/surg patient rooms are initially crowded with medical personnel from multidisciplinary teams (nursing, respiratory, infection control, various physician specialists, pharmacy, nutrition, etc) who are assessing each new patient and recommending a plan of care. Trained personnel come to screen each new patient for any sign of TBI. Conversation is constant, clinical decisions are being made, and changes are taking place. Pain management is a primary concern for patients who have traveled long hours on an uncomfortable litter and are experiencing increased discomfort. Nurses juggle multiple priorities at one time. They are quickly trying to obtain orders for pain medication, swab wounds to rule out multidrug-resistant organisms, complete the enormous volume of required documentation, answer patient questions, and offer continual support. Although addressing patient health is the nurses' first priority issue, personal hygiene is the top concern for many soldiers who have just arrived from the desert. They want to feel clean and refreshed, and wash away the gritty feeling from sand and stale blood from their injuries.[5]

Nurses with various clinical backgrounds have deployed to LRMC. Some arrived having worked in labor and delivery, pediatrics, and outpatient clinics. Seasoned med/surg nurses were invaluable mentors in teaching skills essential to treating casualties of war, such as tracheotomy care, irrigation, dressing changes, and wound care. Patients typically had already undergone at least one surgery in the combat hospital. Wound assessment began on arrival at LRMC, and nurses moved quickly in preparing patients for washout surgery, and then stabilizing them for evacuation to CONUS for further evaluation and treatment. In any given 24-hour period during the height of the war, nursing staff on a med/surg floor might discharge ten patients and admit eleven new ones. This was the typical high-paced, operational tempo that went on day after day at LRMC.

Meeting Additional Needs

Nurses at LRMC have a deep understanding that there are important emotional needs for these wounded warriors, in addition to their physical needs. Once initial medical priorities have been addressed, nurses facilitate calls to family and friends at home. This is the best "support medicine" soldiers can receive. The transfer of patients from combat zone to LRMC happens quickly and efficiently, before many soldiers can ask questions or come to terms with what has happened to them. They are often worried about their units and want to return to duty as soon as possible. Communication with the appropriate chain of command is part of the LRMC protocol, and this is reinforced to soldiers. Amid all of the orders and necessary medical care, nurses do their best to offer as much emotional support to their patients as possible. Many patients are young and have never been hospitalized before. They are often scared and overwhelmed by the entire process. Others need someone to listen and answer questions.

Nurses utilize the supportive resources at LRMC to bolster morale and help meet patient needs, such as obtaining items from the Chaplain's Closet (DVDs, clothes, candy, snacks, books, etc) and making sure each patient returns home with a Quilt of Valor (see Chapter 9, Chaplain Services). Patients also receive a money voucher to purchase clothes, shoes, and other essential items.

IMPLEMENTATION: NURSE CASE MANAGERS
Outpatient Nurse Case Managers

In the early morning, outpatient NCMs pass through the main entrance of the Deployed Warrior Medical Management Center (DWMMC) and stop to scan the mounted flat-screen television that lists the number of expected flights for the day and their anticipated arrival times. This mode of communication is a few notches up the technology ladder compared to the dry erase board used prior to 2010 that had to be updated every evening. Although clinic hours don't begin until 0800, NCMs arrive by 0700, frequently grab whatever coffee they can find, and use this administrative hour to check on details of arriving flights and incoming manifests to learn what patients to expect and their various injuries or illnesses. Patients en route have already been assigned to a particular inpatient or outpatient service by the on-call provider the night before arrival. NCMs glean additional information from the PMRs and electronic outpatient notes (AHLTA [Armed Forces Health Longitudinal Technology Application]) so they know as much as possible before the patient is sitting in front of them in the outpatient NCM office.

The arrival of wounded warriors impacts another group of essential nursing personnel at LRMC. Outpatient NCMs fall under the administrative umbrella of the DWMCC, an integral unit created in 2001 to provide administrative and medical management to US service members evacuated from theater. The DWMMC is located in four bi-level trailers adjacent to the outside entrance of the hospital's emergency department. One of those trailers is home to the NCMs and consists of several small offices where patients are seen. There is also a patient waiting area nicknamed the "fish tank room" because it houses two large freshwater fish tanks. This room is also used for staff to discuss incoming patient briefs.

When the AMBUS pulls up in front of the emergency department, NCMs are often among the group to welcome new patients and assist as needed. After the critically ill soldiers are transported off the AMBUS and immediately taken to the ICU or the med/surg floor, attention turns to the outpatient soldiers. They initially meet with their respective Liaison Noncommissioned Officer (LNO), who provides a personal briefing, identifies any initial needs, and offers support. Every outpatient must be seen by the NCM within 48 hours of arrival time at LRMC. Patients sometimes come directly to see the NCM after their meeting with the LNO, though some may not be seen for a day or two after arrival; that decision typically depends on the severity of their illness/injury and how much instructional information they are able to retain. Often, soldiers miss some of the information given to them because of hearing loss from improvised explosive device blasts. Others are in pain or just not feeling well. All of these soldiers have just traveled on a long flight on a C-17, and are often exhausted, hungry, and uncomfortable. Some have been waiting days for a flight in stopover places like Bagram, Kuwait, or Qatar. Should a patient not report within the specified time, NCMs know which LNO to contact. They are also given the patient's room number at the Medical Transient Detachment and can check on them there.

DWMMC case managers are registered nurses who coordinate outpatient care for wounded warriors and civilians. They work closely with physicians, command liaisons, the service member's command unit, and the DWMMC. Located adjacent to the emergency department, the DWMMC outpatient clinic is the patient's source for primary care, sick visits, medication refills, and TBI screening. NCMs ensure that patients see the correct medical specialist and complete the blood work and medical tests listed on the provider treatment plan. All service members arriving at LRMC from downrange must have a TBI screen completed prior to returning to duty or transferring for continued care. This helps identify those patients who need further neurological services. NCMs also refer patients for additional evaluation if any new concerns are identified during encounters. Although there are multiple specialty outpatient services, the busiest are general surgery and orthopedics. If LRMC does not have the capability to perform certain procedures, patients are sent to a German hospital, usually the Saarland University Medical Center in Homburg, about 30 km west of Landstuhl. Each outpatient must report back to the NCM following every specialty appointment to ensure that all consults are complete. Many soldiers come with sports injuries unrelated to combat injuries.

The NCM is responsible for:
- generating a weekly report to maintain patient flow visibility in accordance with theater evacuation policy;
- entering outpatient encounters in AHLTA (outpatient electronic medical records); and
- entering patient information into the Theater Medical Data Store (TMDS) system to facilitate a seamless and paperless flow of medical information to the next level of care.

Each military branch manages and coordinates outpatient medical care, and patients are followed accordingly:
- Army and Air Force patients are managed by DWMMC NCMs and Army/Air Force LNOs;

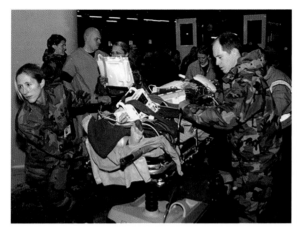

Nurses move quickly while transporting patients from the ambulance bus into Landstuhl Regional Medical Center.

Photograph courtesy of Landstuhl Regional Medical Center.

- Navy and Marine Corps patients do not visit DWMMC NCMs—the Navy LNO coordinates and manages all patient care-related issues; and
- other (Department of Defense civilian, contractor, and foreign national) patients are not managed by DWMMC NCMs (they are managed by the Patient Administrative Division)—inpatient NCMs sometimes become heavily involved with civilians and contractors because of their varying needs and medical insurance.

The average outpatient length of stay at LRMC is 10 days.[6] For that time period, wounded warriors can rely on their NCM as their healthcare advocate. In addition to the responsibilities of managing and coordinating care, NCMs are an invaluable resource and source of support for many soldiers who need someone who cares to listen to what they have seen and been through. As the intensity of the war decreased, staffing needs across the hospital were reduced accordingly. Between 2010 and 2012, there were six outpatient NCMs, which was decreased to four by the fall of 2012, and three in August 2013.

Inpatient Nurse Case Managers

The role of the inpatient NCM at LRMC was initiated in mid-2010 in direct response to the need for improved management of patient care. Trauma to multiple organs and sensory systems necessitated immense coordination of a multitude of specialty services. The continuous flow of critically ill patients evacuated from downrange, and the quick turn-around of patients transferred to CONUS medical treatment facilities (MTFs), required an additional layer of strategic care planning. Lack of coordination during transitions often caused delays and complications for both the patients and the medical staff. Case management therefore became a pivotal role in ensuring continuity of care and keeping track of the whole treatment picture. The goal of inpatient NCMs at LRMC is to optimize patient outcomes, optimize quality of care, and manage costs. Inpatient NCMs report to LRMC's deputy chief of nursing. At the time the role was initiated, the NCM group was comprised of the chief of medical management and five NCMs assigned to specific departments throughout the hospital.

The day begins early for the inpatient NCM who participates in morning multidisciplinary rounds, both in the ICU and on the med/surg floors. When a new patient is admitted to LRMC, NCMs immediately initiate a treatment care plan. Inpatient NCMs are responsible for other patients in their designated area, in addition to wounded warriors, such as those in active duty within the European theater, retirees, and beneficiaries. Goals are initially established based on a thorough patient assessment by various members of the medical team, which helps to identify additional necessary resources. Coordination with various specialists—such as occupational therapy, physical therapy, speech therapy, pharmacy, nutrition, and other medical specialists—begins immediately to ensure early referral to the appropriate teams.

NCMs communicate directly with patients, families (when possible), clinical providers, TRICARE, and other health insurance companies. They are proactive and utilize the nursing process to continually assess the needs of patients and their support systems, facilitate implementation, and evaluate progress. Flexibility is essential because adjustments are often necessary throughout the duration of hospitalization, illness, disability, or need for service. The initial care plan and goals are often readjusted based on clinical and logistical changes and needs. Achieving the best possible patient outcomes and maintaining quality care are balanced with ensuring that available resources are used in a timely and cost-effective manner. NCMs help relieve administrative burdens placed on the providers and patients that could result in delays in patient treatment, recovery, transition to another level of care, or discharge.

Given the extensive and complex injuries sustained by many of the casualties admitted to LRMC, it is paramount to anticipate and plan for the multiple layers of specialty needs. It would not be unusual for any one patient to need the services of seven different specialists as part of his or her treatment and rehabilitation.[7] Discharge planning is therefore initiated at the time of admission to foster the continuation of care. For patients being transferred to CONUS, the NCM ensures that all necessary paperwork is in order and disseminated to the proper departments. Planning for successful transitional care is another important element of case management. Transition of care takes place when patients move between care settings, return home, go to a rehabilitation facility, or experience a change in medical status or personal situation. Lack of coordination during these transitions can cause delays and complications for everyone involved. Successful transitions involve extensive coordination between the patients, clinical and administrative staff at LRMC, the receiving MTF, the Theater Patient Movement Requirement Center, and the Global Patient Movement Requirement Center. NCMs also ensure that the families of wounded soldiers have been contacted and that updates are routinely communicated to the appropriate chain of command. This level of care and detail for a caseload of wounded soldiers requires a high degree of organization and a strong clinical skill set.

Inpatient NCMs also participate in weekly multidisciplinary patient care conferences to collaborate and coordinate services and plan discharges. Nurse and physician representatives from each unit and various specialty services attend these weekly meetings, and provide input on the specific needs of each patient. Each inpatient is reviewed, and those with a significant change in status, or needing additional care or services beyond what they are currently receiving, are discussed. Adjustments to care plans are made according to how the patient is progressing and whether the established goals can be attained by discharge. When possible, patients and family members may attend these conferences. Bi-monthly guest speakers give presentations at the conferences on a variety of relevant topics to educate staff, promote professional growth, and decrease fragmentation of care. All patient care conferences and related decisions are summarized in the patient's inpatient medical records.

Each NCM at LRMC is knowledgeable about the hospital's clinical guidelines, standard operating procedures, and protocols. NCMs often are responsible for briefing the continually rotating staff, which is particularly essential at LRMC due to the constant turnover from multiple deployments and reassignments.

LESSONS LEARNED

It is almost inconceivable when one thinks about the multiple levels of care that occur for a casualty who is first treated with a tourniquet to stop the bleeding in the combat field and later arrives at LRMC. Yet this complex care happened, day after day, hour after hour, and with a great deal of success. More than 90,000 wounded warriors from Afghanistan and Iraq have been treated at LRMC as they made their way through the medical evacuation system and back home.[8] Severely ill or injured critical care patients typically arrive in Germany after one or more operations in the last 24 to 36 hours, and will likely require another operation within 3 to 12 hours after arrival. This surgery will be done by a surgeon different from the one who performed the primary surgery and different from the surgeon who will perform any necessary future surgeries in CONUS. Patients have survived the initial procedures, and have just traveled 5 to 10 hours at an altitude greater than 30,000 feet, at an ambient pressure of half an atmosphere,

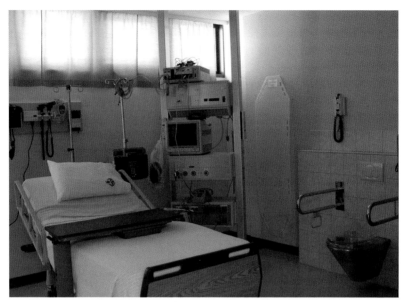

Patient care area in the intensive care unit at Landstuhl Regional Medical Center.
Photograph courtesy of CDR Kevin Kumlien, Navy reservist, Intensive Care Unit nurse.

strapped to a stretcher, and receiving continuous high-level critical care en route.[9] Most clinicians would agree that these same critically ill patients would not be considered stable enough to move from a civilian ICU to have a CT scan, yet they have just been moved from a combat hospital to a plane and traveled multiple hours, and are moved again.

Electronic medical records from downrange have preceded approximately 80% of the patients that arrive. The rest of the time, information is written on surgical wound dressings, passed on by the CCATT team, or both. In either case, clinicians would agree this is more information than what they get from patients who arrive off the street in US trauma centers. The critical care team at LRMC interviews the CCATT team about the patient's condition during the flight to verify the accuracy and completeness of all information. Once settled in the hospital, each patient is then reassessed with a complete history and detailed physical examination as if the patient had not been seen before.[9] All of this takes place at LRMC at the same time hospital staff are continuing quality primary care and inpatient care to the 450,000 military personnel stationed in Europe, southwest Asia, and Africa.[5]

People are the lifeline in any organization, mission, or goal. The extraordinary measures described herein could only have occurred because of the extraordinary individuals making them happen. Nurses were a vital part of this remarkable team who worked relentlessly to care for wounded warriors for those few days that they were patients at LRMC, and then sent home or returned to duty. Although most people would agree that the rewards were beyond words and the experience would be a part of them forever, there was a price that came with that commitment. Care for the caregiver was a vital lesson learned and a necessary part of this human endeavor that took place at LRMC. The invaluable contribution of nursing to the GWOT cannot be forgotten.

Successes

- *Dedication to quality care.* The nurses who served their country at LRMC during the GWOT left an impeccable trail of dedication, hard work, and the highest quality of care. They pushed aside their own exhaustion, stress, homesickness, and grief to do what was needed. Despite the despair they themselves felt from the devastating injuries they witnessed day after day, they put a smile on their faces for their patients. Every measure was taken to provide an optimal level of care for these brave men and women who were now wounded warriors. Nurses were compelled by their own desire to do their best, push their limits in the face of extremely challenging circumstances, and provide exceptional care for their patients who sacrificed so much in the name of freedom. They helped train each other, advocated for patient needs, and worked together for the common mission. The nurses at LRMC set a high standard of care for the modern hospital battlefield. A deployed trauma surgeon and a visiting civilian vascular surgeon both remarked that "great nursing care kept these patients alive" (telephone interviews with Colonel Warren Dorlac, former medical director, Trauma and Critical Care, LRMC; September 2014, and Dr. Michael S. Weingarten, civilian vascular surgeon; December 2014). To these clinicians, who had both witnessed and treated the repercussions of the war, it was atrocity at its worst and humanity at its best.

- *Internal support.* During work hours, nurses took care of their patients. When the shift was over, they did the best they could to support and take care of each other as friends and substitute families. They laughed and cried together. No one other than coworkers could understand the enormity of what they experienced on a daily basis. People coped in various ways just to survive the sadness. There was no judgment, only understanding from those who were doing their best to cope. Hospital chaplains also provided an important support system as they encouraged staff to recognize and accept all of their feelings, good and bad. They listened, advised, validated, and grieved with caretakers, recognizing the toll their jobs were taking on their emotional and physical health. All medical staff was encouraged to volunteer on the chaplain day trips, which took ambulatory soldiers sightseeing to local areas and for meals in German restaurants. These trips were supported by private donations and brought a great deal of benefit to both patient and professional. It was therapeutic for staff to see patients out of uniform, relaxing, having fun, and enjoying life. This renewed their sense of hope and reinforced the value of the work they did so tirelessly.

- *Collaboration of nurse teams.* The military trauma transport system had its own unique challenges based on the rapid movement of critically ill patients from several MTFs, evaluation and treatment by multiple providers, and travel across three continents and multiple time zones. The likelihood for some degree of miscommunication was inevitable given the complexities of this large, multitiered system. The ongoing collaboration among trauma nurse coordinators and all unit-specific nurses within the Joint Theater Trauma System (JTTS) facilitated communication and provided the much needed consistency to ensure continuum of care.[5]

- *Performance improvement.* Performance improvement (PI) and evaluation of critical care were among the greatest successes in the treatment of wounded warriors. Before a patient even arrived at LRMC, all members of the healthcare team could monitor and track medical records and trauma activation and compliance with clinical guidelines by viewing the Joint Patient Tracking Application. One of the greatest successful examples of this was the JTTS Burn Clinical Management Guideline.[10] A burn flow sheet was developed to efficiently communicate ongoing fluid resuscitation as the patient moved across the evacuation continuum of care from several providers and hospitals, spanning three continents and several time zones.[10] This continuous means of communication significantly improved patient outcomes, with decreased abdominal compartment syndrome and decreased mortality.[11] The trauma nurse coordinator was also responsible for monitoring the trauma registry database that tracked all PI issues. Any complication identified was conveyed to the clinical nurses and providers, and appropriate changes were made to the patient's plan of care.

Nurses also participated in a unique PI process through a weekly video teleconference (VTC), including members of the trauma team across the entire evacuation spectrum of care, from field hospitals in the combat zone, to LRMC, to four stateside MTFs that received patients during OEF/OIF. During the VTCs, discussions were held on transport and equipment, clinical care, complications, improving outcomes, and communication. A monthly JTTS VTC was held specifically to focus on optimizing nursing care. Teleconferencing proved invaluable in addressing problematic issues, ensuring standards of care, improving communication, and improving patient care across the board.[5]

Challenges

- *Patient population.* The demographics of the LRMC patient population changed drastically with the onset of the GWOT. During peacetime, the average age of patients was over 50 years, and typical diagnoses included heart and lung disease, stroke, complications from diabetes, gastrointestinal bleeding, and the need for general surgery. After the beginning of OEF/OIF, the patient landscape looked very different: the average age dropped from 18 to 24 years, and primary diagnoses now included polytrauma, burns, amputations, penetrating wounds, and open and closed-head injuries. This sudden shift in demographics caused a roller coaster of emotions for nurses, who saw these young men and women as someone's spouse, parent, son or daughter, and friend. The realization that these young lives were changed forever by disfigurement, TBI, and deep emotional scars was extremely painful. There was also the realization that many of these service members had young families at home whose lives were now changed forever. It was emotional listening to wounded warriors tell their families, "I am coming home, but just different than when I left."[5] Patients came and went quickly, and nurses often worried and wondered how they adjusted and coped once they were back home and the realities of their injuries and the implications for their lives set in.

> *One of my biggest challenges is not having closure with the patients I cared for after they left Landstuhl. We always hear if the patients did not make it, but not always the stories about their recovery progress. You cannot help but think about what happened to the patients, how the families are doing, etc. I have to find peace for myself, knowing that we got them "home," knowing that the excellent medical care and medical personnel commitment will see them through at the other military hospitals. Still, I would like to know how they are doing.*
>
> — DEE DEE PRICE, CIVILIAN ICU NURSE, LRMC

- *Compassion fatigue.* The hospital nursing care and inpatient/outpatient nurse case management at LRMC were of the highest caliber. The level of commitment and dedication to quality care never wavered. Yet the critical injuries, demanding workload, young patients, staff turnover, and distance from family and friend support brought significant stress to caretakers and took a toll. This increased stress level was characterized as *secondary traumatization* or *compassion fatigue*.[12] Symptoms are similar to those of posttraumatic stress disorder (PTSD) and can range from difficulty sleeping, anxiety, depression, anger, fear, and grief to lack of motivation, feeling overwhelmed, cognitive problems, and physical fatigue. Nurses look at their patients and see young lives just beginning and now changed forever. They heard about pregnant wives at home giving birth while their husbands were diagnosed with severe TBI.[12] Nurses were also dealing with problems and stress in their personal lives because many left spouses and children at home when they deployed. As work pressures accumulated, there was less ability to cope and a higher incidence of symptoms. Those nurses with grief or stress prior to deployment were at highest risk for developing PTSD-type problems.

- *High turnover and diversity in nursing staff.* The unique nursing environment of LRMC itself added another dimension to the various challenges and stress of caring for critically ill and injured soldiers. This diverse group consists of active duty and reserve nurses from the Army, Navy, and Air Force, as well as civilian nurses hired through the Department of Defense. In most instances, these nurses were given little notice before deployment to a foreign country a continent away. Despite the differences across military branches, the nurses joined forces as dedicated professionals caring for wounded warriors. However, challenges arose in the constant turnover of staff. Typically, active duty nurses are assigned for 2 to 3 years, whereas reservists are assigned to LRMC for 1 year. Sometimes, these reservists were at LRMC for only 2 to 3 weeks and then were reassigned. In addition, some active duty nurses were assigned to other external military units in addition to LRMC. This meant they might leave the hospital for days to weeks at a time for specialized training in the field, leaving gaps in nursing support that increased the workload for those who remained behind. Some Air Force nurses were also part of the medical evacuation team and could be called upon at any time to transport patients out of the country. They, too, might be gone for days at a time. This constant flux in staff numbers and turnover caused a level of chaos, stress, and heavy workload that was a perpetual challenge.[5]

- *Training.* Nurses come to LRMC with a variety of clinical backgrounds. The nature of complex injuries due to the destructive forms of combat in Iraq and Afghanistan required a high level of medical and trauma care. Nurses in civilian hospitals were used to practicing in a certain specialty area; however, nurses at LRMC needed to know how to care for a multitrauma patient who needed a multitude of specialists, such as orthopedics, neurology, pulmonary, and burn care. Although military nursing has always maintained high standards of care reflecting evidence-based practice, the constant turnover of nursing staff with different types of training made the consistent implementation of this practice a constant challenge.

- *Burn care.* When nurses arrived at LRMC, they were typically assigned to units that matched their skill level, experience, education, and competency. Most ICU nurses at LRMC worked in other ICU settings in either other military or civilian hospitals. Most had some trauma experience, albeit nothing to the extent of what they experienced at LRMC. However, most did not have burn care experience, which is typically its own specialty unit or hospital in the US medical system. Many wounded soldiers arrived in the ICU and the med/surg units with various degrees of burns. Wound care was essential, as well as identifying the clinical risks of burn patients. Most nurses wished that they had more experience and training in this specialty. They relied on their strong clinical instincts, and for a period of time, on the expertise of a civilian nurse with burn care experience.

During my first three years in the ICU at LRMC, the war in Iraq brought a higher percentage of burn patients. My preceptor was previously stationed at the BAMC [Brooke Army Medical Center, Fort Sam Houston] burn unit; thus burn care became my specialty. Our burn patients were always 60% to 95% TBSA [total body surface area] burns. Multi-trauma patients arrived with opened abdomens, fractures with ex-fixes, head injuries, and/ or burns. From 2004 to 2007, we would have up to 20 to 24 vented multi- trauma patients, and at one point eight burn patients arrived on one flight.
— DEE DEE PRICE, CIVILIAN ICU NURSE, LRMC

- *Reintegration.* Caregivers, like soldiers, find it difficult to reintegrate after deployment. There is a feeling of "not fitting in" once they reenter the civilian world. Although reuniting with family is wonderful, it often brings stress and uncertainty. Some deployed caregivers find it difficult to talk about what their experience was like and how they were impacted. They are not sure anyone could understand what they went through unless they were there to see and live it firsthand. Others learn that family and friends do not want to hear about their experiences and find it hard to relate to a world thousands of miles away. Spouses often felt alone and resented handling all the responsibilities of home and children while the other partner was away. Divorce and separation rates after deployments are relatively high. Deployed personnel have to learn to reacclimate and figure out where they fit in. Those who return to work in their civilian jobs learn that their positions were held by other individuals in their absence. This transition is often awkward for coworkers as more changes are then made. Additional support and attention are essential for these exceptional caregivers in helping them to reintegrate and return to civilian life. They have made great sacrifices and contributed a valuable service to their country. They are often in a vulnerable state, and it is paramount to recognize and respond to their unique needs.

My first burn patient who passed away in 2006 was a young soldier, 95% burn patient, who starting coding within 15 minutes after he was in my room. There were only a few people in the room—the anesthesiologist, the respiratory therapist, myself, two trauma attending physicians, and one other nurse with the medications. We did everything we could to try to save him; his injuries were just too significant.

When I returned to LRMC in 2008, I had two patients pass away within 2 days of each other. The first patient was a young marine with a high amputation. Most people do not know that not too many families are at LRMC, due to the high turnaround of our patients to the states, yet the parents of both of these patients were at their bedsides. The marine's family was at his bedside when he passed, and I found some comfort knowing his mom and dad were able to be there with him. The second patient was a 90% burn patient. My coworker and I came to work about 0300 to receive a flight with two burn patients. I had a second nurse helping me because I did the burn care with the physician. We stayed for over 17 hours that day. He passed within 2 hours of my arrival at work the next day. His mother was at his bedside that day. She kept telling me thank you, thank you for trying to save him. She hugged me. I remember feeling numb, and I sat on the floor of the next patient's room and just cried. The service members I have taken care of still affect me to this day and always bring tears that I/we could not fix or save them all. I always thought, if I can just get them home to their families, they will be okay. It was when we could not that affected me the most.

— DEE DEE PRICE, CIVILIAN ICU NURSE, LRMC

ACKNOWLEDGMENTS

The authors thank CDR Lisa Lewis, Navy Reservist, outpatient NCM; CDR Kevin Kumlien, Navy Reservist, ICU nurse; CDR Pamela Patnode, Navy Reservist, Medical/Surgical nurse; Dee Dee Price, civilian ICU nurse; CAPT Mary Norgaard, Navy Reservist, Medical/Surgical nurse; Jane Darigo, civilian outpatient NCM; and Kathryn Gillespie, civilian, Chief Inpatient NCM.

REFERENCES

1. US Army. Army Medicine: Landstuhl Regional Medical Center website. http://www.goarmy.com/amedd/health-care/facilities/landstuhl-regional-medical-center.html. Accessed November 23, 2015.
2. Dorland P, Nanney J. *Dust Off: Army Aeromedical Evacuation in Vietnam.* Washington, DC: Center of Military History; 2008: 4.
3. Robbins S. Landstuhl staff busy as Afghan fight intensifies. *Stars and Stripes.* November 13, 2009.
4. Grills M. Out of harm's way. *The American Legion Magazine.* March 1, 2008.
5. Steele N, Katz A, Martin K, Garcia D, Womble S, Wright H. Rewards and challenges of nursing wounded warriors at Landstuhl Regional Medical Center, Germany. *Nurs Clin North Am.* 2010;45(2):205–218.
6. *Fact Sheet–Deployed Warrior Medical Management Center, Landstuhl Regional Medical Center.* Landstuhl, Germany: LRMC Public Affairs Office; July 2009.
7. Cobbs A, Pidgen N. Polytrauma care: a delicate balance for the military nurse case manager. *J Trauma Nurs.* 2008;15(4):192–196.
8. *Fact Sheet–Landstuhl Regional Medical Center.* Landstuhl, Germany: LRMC Public Affairs Office; September 2015.
9. McSwain N. Musings from Landstuhl Regional Medical Center. After Action Report, July 8–30, 2007. http://www.aast.org/Assets/b94716d3-8178-4a69-bb1c-147fb9bd3530/633870595881200000/after-action-report-final-v9-16-pdf. Accessed November 15, 2015.
10. Chung LL, Blackbourne LH, Wolf SE. Evolution of burn resuscitation in Operation Iraqi Freedom. *J Burn Care Res.* 2006;27(5):606–611.
11. Holcomb JB, McMulin NR, Pearse L. Causes of death in U.S. Special Operations Forces in the global war on terrorism: 2001–2004. *Ann Surg.* 2007;245(6):986–991; Abstract.
12. Kenny D. Critical care nurses' experiences caring for the casualties of war evacuated from the front lines: lessons learned and needs identified. *Crit Care Nurs Clin North Am.* 2008;20(1):41–49.

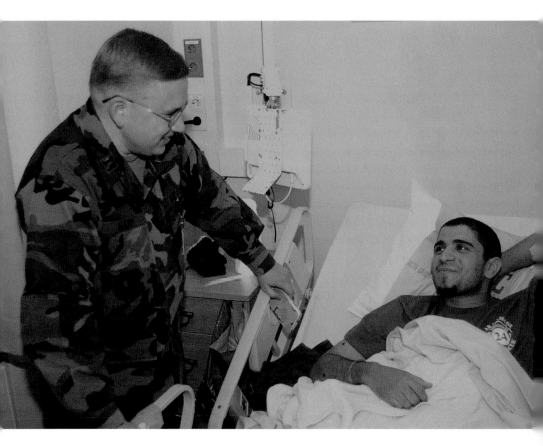

Chaplain at bedside visiting with a wounded warrior.

CHAPTER NINE

Chaplain Services

"Pro Deo et Patria" (For God and Country)

*Where does one ever find the right words to comfort a soldier who has lost
two limbs, a soldier who is the only remaining survivor from his mission, or a
nurse cradling a 19-year old in her arms while he draws his last breath?
What do you say to a family who has flown 10 hours across oceans to say
good-bye to their son or daughter, child before soldier, who once romped in
overalls before camouflage? Is there enough faith to offer a surgeon, on his feet in
an operating room for 48 hours, called upon to exercise his mastered craft,
while making decisions that change the lives of the human beings entrusted
to his care? There are no "right words," cards, platitudes, or phrases to fill the
vacant hole occupied by a sadness and despair chronically lingering in the
shadows of such realities. This was daily life at Landstuhl Regional
Medical Center starting in 2001.*

oldiers come into the military with diverse religious backgrounds, some
with none at all. Faith is personal, individual, and predictably changeable
with the natural ebb and flow of life events. Like nature's seasons, faith
experiences dreary winters, hearts barren as naked trees, and glorious springs,
hearts bursting with blooming color and radiant hope. Faith can be tumultuous,
snapping with emotions as vivid as an autumn day strewn with fiery red and burnt
orange leaves swirling the air on their descent to the ground. Like a lazy breeze
on a summer day, faith can also be lackadaisical, paying little attention to time or
commitment. There are likely few life events that could shake the foundation of
one's faith more than war. It takes great inner strength to cope with the magnitude
of loss that barrels forward in every direction. In a split second, a life can be lost
or changed forever. What can really prepare the human psyche to cope with the
depth and breadth of the physical and emotional suffering that war brings . . . to a
soldier, a caretaker, a family, or an entire nation?

Military chaplains have always been a source of comfort and strength for men and women in the armed services, especially during war.[1] They help soldiers cope with the overwhelming circumstances they encounter, such as: combat stress, environmental challenges, separation from family and friends, and physical and emotional loss. The chaplains at Landstuhl Regional Medical Center (LRMC) are an integral part of the war effort and have greatly impacted the lives of soldiers, staff, and family members. Their mission is as follows: *The Clinical Pastoral Division at LRMC provides religious and counseling support to the military community, staff, and patients. The staff of Air Force, Army, and Navy personnel consists of active duty, Guard and Reserve chaplains and chaplain assistants, as well as full-time civilians and volunteers.*[2]

BACKGROUND

Prior to the onset of Operation Iraqi Freedom and Operation Enduring Freedom, LRMC functioned primarily as an American-based community hospital. Until September 2001, it was staffed with two chaplains and two chaplain assistants. Fast forward to 2004, when time unfolded to a completely different story: a community hospital turned trauma center, now staffed with thirteen chaplains and seven chaplain assistants. The changes in wartime intensity brought changes to the chaplain role as well. No longer was it a matter of only visiting patients and making notes as needed. Chaplains rotated shifts because they were required to be on-call 24 hours a day. Documentation on every patient seen was now mandatory. Chaplains were required to meet all incoming flights from Ramstein upon arrival at LRMC, regardless of time of day or night. Uncertainty was the only "certainty" they could truly count on because there was no consistent schedule for flight arrivals, suffering, or death.

Military chaplains require a high level of training and experience prior to entering the military. They must have a graduate degree in theology, have a minimum of 2 years of professional experience, and be considered a qualified leader in their particular religious denomination. At the time of application, they undergo a physical examination and security clearance. Although they are non-combatants, they still undergo a type of military training. For example, the Army requires chaplains to attend the Chaplain Basic Officer Leadership Course, which provides an introduction to noncombatant core skills.[3]

In addition, hospitals then require military chaplains to complete a 1-year Clinical Pastoral Education (CPE) course. The military CPE program is one of the most effective chaplain training environments for battlefield ministry.[4] Topics during the training include crisis counseling, death and dying, grief counseling, family systems, and spirituality. There are also a variety of seminars that focus on reflection, worship, and interpersonal relationships. Throughout the year, there is supervisory one-on-one training and consultation for pastoral education, and regular annual and monthly training provided for most chaplains.

IMPLEMENTATION

The chaplain is the first person who meets wounded warriors right off the ambulance bus when they arrive at LRMC. From that point on, there are multiple duties and responsibilities throughout the day. Chaplains provide religious services for a variety of faiths, make daily bedside visits to all sick and injured inpatients, including both wounded warriors and local civilian patients, and spend time with outpatient soldiers. Wounded warriors, civilian contractors, and coalition troops come from a total of 44 different countries treated at LRMC.[2]

One of the most integral roles for the chaplain is that of counselor. There is a great deal of physical and emotional suffering in wartime. Loss is a continual theme. Chaplains help wounded warriors come to terms with and make sense of their traumatic experiences. The pastoral staff also monitor the emotional thermometer of the caretakers at LRMC, who deal with trauma and high stress on a continual basis.

Chaplain Ronald Pettigrew is a soft-spoken man. His smile is warm and wide and engages you immediately; his words, even more so. The soft-spoken voice speaks with conviction, passion, and truth about the devastation wounded warriors have faced, the impact on their families, the toll on caretakers, and what it means to experience this on a daily basis at LRMC. Humanity and compassion mingle with his honesty. Ronald Pettigrew has an unwavering belief in the goodness of his God, which likely explains his aura of tranquility and an acceptance of what is. Although suffering often lures people into an emotional tug-of-war between what is fair and what is not, Pettigrew has somehow moved past the point of questioning "why" and focuses instead on "what more can we do?"

Chaplain Pettigrew, a Navy Reservist, has been deployed twice to LRMC; the first time in 2006–2007 and again in 2012. The second time, his wife and daughters came to Germany with him. Although this was an initial adjustment for them with new work, school, and friends, keeping the family together was worth the changes. There was an additional intention with this decision as well. Although both parents felt it was enriching for their children to live in another county and experience another culture, the decision was deeper than even that. It was a way for Pettigrew's children to see and feel the value and meaning of daily life at LRMC, the reason for their father's role, and a way to understand commitment to one's country. On a personal level, he and his family felt blessed.

On a professional level, the chaplain is continually humbled. His patients are his best teachers on what is important in life. He considers each moment and conversation he shares with a soldier to be a privilege. Chaplain Pettigrew is continually amazed by the selfless attitude of each wounded warrior who arrives at LRMC. No matter the extent of their injuries, they are more concerned with others rather than themselves. He is amazed by these young men and women, some of them still teenagers, who understand that they are part of something bigger than themselves. He gives an example of this when he talks about his initial visits with soldiers and repeatedly hears the same questions from all of them:

- "Where's my Sergeant?"
- "When can I return to my unit?"
- "Did [name of comrade] make it?"
- If someone did not make it, they ask, "How can I take care of his or her family?"

There is also consistency in the painful issues faced by wounded warriors:

- survivor's guilt,
- separation anxiety (from their unit),
- grief, and
- denial.

The nature of recent wars has resulted in insidious injuries, and often soldiers arrive at LRMC having lost one or more limbs. The chaplain sees that many are initially in denial when hearing of their injuries. Often, they will instead focus on getting back to their respective units. It takes a while to absorb the enormity of the news and the impact this new reality will have on their lives.

Chaplain Pettigrew recalls a story of a solider in the intensive care unit who was a quadriplegic as a result of his injuries. It was initially difficult for him to speak, and he did not want to talk to a chaplain. Pettigrew used a message board and moved letters up and down to communicate with the soldier, who eventually, over time, opened up with his feelings. The soldier's wife had made several attempts to call and talk to him, but he was afraid to talk to her. He expressed his fears and worries about providing for his family due to his injuries. Never once did he ever really worry about himself. Chaplain Pettigrew contacted the soldier's wife and put the soldier on the phone. Over and over again, she reiterated to him how much she loved him and that she was not going anywhere. She cried and told him she was just so happy he was alive and could come home to their family. After the conversation, the soldier spelled out the word "R-I-N-G" on the message board. He wanted to wear his wedding ring.

Stories and experiences such as this were the victories that kept him going, but Ronald Pettigrew is honest to also say that there were many hard days as well. He admits to feeling helpless at times. Was he doing enough? What would happen to these soldiers when they left LRMC? Was there enough available support for them in their process of grieving and adjusting?

Chaplain Pettigrew has experienced firsthand the power of human connection. As simple as that sounds, it may be the most significant ingredient in a soldier's recovery. Both big and small efforts work concomitantly in making a difference. What he also saw firsthand was the generosity of the human heart, especially the American heart. Programs such as the Chaplain's Closet (see Saying Thank You . . . One Box at a Time: The Chaplain's Closet) and the Quilts of Valor (see Saying Thank You . . . One Stitch at a Time: The Quilts of Valor Foundation) were born out of the sheer effort and determination of two American military spouses/mothers who saw a need and wanted to help. Their impact has been far-reaching, as volunteers around the country have been inspired by their spirit and have joined in supporting their mission. Chaplain Pettigrew has seen how this trickle-down effect, from a small American town to the bedside at LRMC, has touched the hearts of wounded warriors. Some have been moved to tears by the generosity of strangers who want them to know how much their sacrifice for their country means. Someone cares; a stranger no less. That fact alone is a powerful tool in the healing process.

Many locals have been bitten by the "need to volunteer bug" and have come forth to help in any way. This includes both American citizens living in Germany, as well as German locals themselves. Hot meals, soda, snacks, and deserts are delivered on a regular basis to the United Service Organization. The chaplain day trips for outpatient wounded warriors are run by the chaplain ministry and supported by volunteers. The bus driver for these trips, who is retired from the Army and living in Germany, is devoted to the ministry. He speaks fluent German and helps pick the best restaurants and interprets as needed. Week after week, he goes out of his way to make sure everyone is comfortable on the bus trips. A grin crosses Chaplain Pettigrew's face when he refers to Marcos, a once perfect stranger, and now a genuine friend.

> *Taking care of these soldiers is as natural for him as breathing. He does not just drive the bus to get us where we want to go. He takes the time to get to know these men and women on a deep and personal level. He likes to chat, and share a soda and a few jokes with them. Marcos believes this is his chance to help take care of their hearts and souls.*

The chaplain day trips are staffed by hospital medical volunteers. Pettigrew sees this as equally beneficial to soldiers and staff. Participating in the trips gives caretakers an opportunity to interact and get to know wounded warriors outside

Saying Thank You . . . One Box at a Time
The Chaplain's Closet

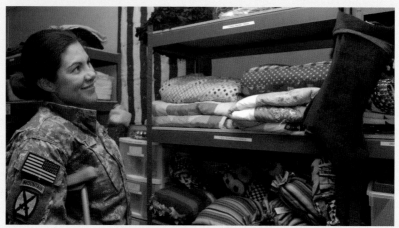

A Christmas stocking and shelves of donated items bring a smile to this soldier.
Photograph courtesy of the Public Affairs Office, Landstuhl Regional Medical Center.

The dictionary defines the word "closet" as a small room or space used for storing things.[1] That is likely not the first impression one gets opening the door to the "Chaplain's Closet" at Landstuhl Regional Medical Center (LRMC). The "closet" is more like the size of a convenience store and supplied with enough stock for a satellite PX (Post Exchange).

The history of this effort dates to October 2001, with the onset of Operation Enduring Freedom. Injured soldiers certainly did not have time to pack their belongings before being flown from the Middle East to Germany for medical care. Many arrived with only the bloody and torn clothing they were wearing at the time of their injuries. If they were lucky, their belongings might have been thrown into a bag, arriving on a different flight. By late 2002, as combat casualties continued to flow into Germany, Landstuhl nurses decided more needed to be done for their patients. It was now winter and wounded warriors were arriving straight from the battlefield without coats, sufficient warm clothing, or personal care items. Provisions were needed until their bags caught up with them from downrange.[2]

The Wounded Warrior Ministry Center began as boxes lined in a hallway with donations from staff, local churches, and charities. The boxes were then stored in an actual closet in the chaplain's office, thus giving origin to the nickname "Chaplain's Closet." Today, there is a large designated room adjacent to the

Pastoral Division that holds these supplies. Overflow boxes are stored in other buildings. Rows and rows of shelves line one part of the Chaplain's Closet, organized by clothing type, color, and size for both men and women. Toiletry items, such as toothbrushes, toothpaste, shampoo, soap, etc, are in a separate section. Ambulatory soldiers come and "shop" for items they need, ranging from sweatpants, T-shirts, underwear, and socks, to athletic shoes, duffel bags, favorite candy, CDs, DVDs, towels, quilts, sheets, phone cards, handheld games, and books. Liaison officers and chaplain staff fill the requested needs of those patients unable to leave their rooms.[3]

As the war progressed, the needs of the Chaplain's Closet quickly surpassed the local donations. In 2004, a very kind and caring American named Karen Grimord came to Germany. She was there visiting her daughter and son-in-law stationed at Ramstein Air Force Base. During that visit, Karen learned from her daughter that LRMC had a very small collection of movies (DVD/VHS) for the wounded soldiers to watch while recuperating from their injuries. Karen returned to the States and got busy putting the word out to her family and friends of this need. They joined efforts with a Boy Scouts group from Huntsville, Alabama, and collected 485 DVDs and VHS tapes to send to the Chaplain's Closet at LRMC.[4]

This donation was met with great enthusiasm and appreciation, so much so that the Landstuhl chaplain asked Karen if she could now collect sweatpants because they were greatly in need. That was all Karen needed to hear, and again she got busy. She turned to family and friends and between all of them came up with 108 donated pairs. The chaplain was again greatly appreciative, but Karen was shocked to learn this number was a "drop in the bucket" to meet the hospital's needs. At the time, as many as 1,000 soldiers were arriving at the hospital every month, and their first stop was the Chaplain's Closet. Supplies were dwindling daily.

Such a reality might have daunted most, but not Karen Grimord. If anyone understood military mission and the needs of soldiers, it was this woman. She entered the world as a military brat, born in a

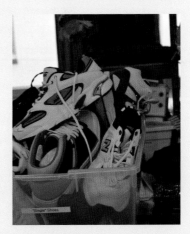

There is something for everyone in the Chaplain's Closet, including a box of single shoes for amputees. No needs go unattended.

Photograph courtesy of the Public Affairs Office, Landstuhl Regional Medical Center.

military hospital, and surrounded by supportive military families her entire life. Both her husband and father served in the Air Force and, at one point, five family members served in the Middle East at the same time. Although it had never been a goal to start a nonprofit organization, Karen moved forward and began the Landstuhl Hospital Care Project. Initially, she used her own money and savings to meet the requests of the perpetual wish list. In the first year, her organization sent out 33 boxes of supplies. But the seesaw of supply and demand continued, and Karen quickly learned that the more supplies she mailed to Landstuhl, the greater the requests for donations. She then reached out to churches, charities, and veterans groups, such as the American Legion, and soon donations came pouring in. Karen also knew she needed help with the legal and financial realities of running a charitable organization. Today, the organization is supported by a small group of volunteers, many with strong military ties, who handle accounting, communications, and other vital support services.[4]

Karen Grimord became known as the "woman from Stafford, Virginia, who could not said no" when it came to a need of a soldier. The two-car garage in the Stafford home is full of boxes, both flat and full. On any given day and at any hour, Karen Grimord is seen sorting through supplies, filling boxes, or taping them shut ready to be sent to those in need. Sometimes there are volunteers, but mostly it is just Karen. She even traded in her beloved Jeep for a Chevy Suburban, better able to handle the volume of her loads and her trips to the post office 4 to 5 days a week.[4]

So what actually goes into these boxes? What are the most popular "hot ticket requests"? Dark clothes are preferred—blacks, grays, and blues. The plainer the better, although one year a large donation of flannel pants with the "Sarge" character from the Pixar/Disney animated film "Cars" was a huge hit. Although soldiers do not like a lot of corporate logos all over their clothes, they do have a sense of humor and Sarge was very popular! Quality is a must. As Karen sifts through the endless piles of stock, she asks herself, "Would I want to wear or use this? A "yes" makes it into the box, and a "no" gets put aside. Smaller, rather than full-size, toiletries are preferred because soldiers may be at LRMC for only a few days. Water bottles, underwear, socks, Crocs, and sneakers of every size are universal needs. Soldiers need diversion and fun, so magazines, books, games, CDs, and DVDs are entertainment essentials. Snacks, candy, and nonperishable food take up valuable space and are greatly appreciated. Everyone needs a treat and a reminder of home.[4]

This extraordinary mission is responsible for shipping more than 200,000 pounds of donated clothes and supplies to wounded warriors. What started as 33 boxes a month is now up to almost 2,000 boxes a month.[4] There is no greater labor of love. Although the majority of donated items are sent to LRMC, Karen

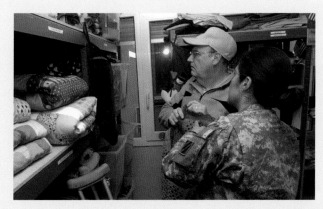

A volunteer at the Chaplain's Closet assists a soldier with making a selection.

Photograph courtesy of the Public Affairs Office, Landstuhl Regional Medical Center.

also sends supplies to medics, nurses, and chaplains at more than 150 military units throughout Afghanistan, Iraq, and other Middle East countries with US military operations.[3]

Perhaps what drives this "Virginia angel" to pack just one more box is her own annual, self-funded trip to Germany, where she volunteers for a month in the Chaplain's Closet at LRMC. Karen Grimord sees firsthand the reactions of soldiers as they receive items of need. She sees a smile of appreciation and a flash of hope simply because these soldiers know that people care about them. Karen also sees firsthand what they have been through. That is enough to get her back on the plane to the States and into her garage to get busy once again.

Americans are known for their generosity and patriotic spirit. This extraordinary humanitarian effort reflects just that. Karen Grimord represents that unified effort to combat the war on terrorism . . . one box at a time.

REFERENCES

1. Merriam-Webster online dictionary. http://www.merriam-webster.com. Accessed April 28, 2015.

2. Landstuhl Regional Medical Center Public Affairs Office. *Fact Sheet–Pastoral Division, Landstuhl Regional Medical Center.* Landstuhl, Germany: LRMC; June 2009.

3. Greenhill J. *Chaplains' closet helps Landstuhl's wounded warriors.* American Forces Press Service. June 26, 2009. http://www.defense.gov/news/newsarticle.aspx?id=54926. Accessed April 28, 2015.

4. Evans JA. American angel. *Saturday Evening Post.* November/Dececember 2012. http://www.saturdayeveningpost.com/2012/11/27/in-the-magazine/people-and-places/american-angel.html. Accessed April 28, 2015.

of the acute setting where intensity and stress are high. It is therapeutic for them to talk and get to know soldiers as themselves, not just as patients who are recovering or facing life-threatening injuries. Soldiers get to know their caretakers as individuals with interests, humor, and personal lives, something that gets forgotten in the business of a hospital setting. The line separating patient from professional erases just a bit on chaplain day trips, where staff dress casually in jeans rather than scrubs and white lab coats. Volunteer hours are supported by hospital administration; staff members are not required to take personal leave. The majority of them return to volunteer again, and they tell the chaplain staff how much these experiences renew their sense of hope and meaning in the work they do at LRMC.

LESSONS LEARNED

The chaplain ministry has played an essential role in supporting wounded warriors, families, and caretakers at LRMC. Soldiers want and need to tell their stories. They need a supportive environment and the right person who responds to a cue to hold a hand, offer a prayer, sit and listen, or simply just sit in silence. They need that person who can absorb and respond to the enormity of their individual suffering, pain, and grief. Whether they choose to connect it to their faith is personal. What is universal, however, is the feeling that their story and experiences are valued. Even in the short amount of time some of the patients are at LRMC, chaplains can quickly identify the various stages of grief as described by Elizabeth Kübler-Ross.[5] Healing is painful. Healing takes time. There are no shortcuts or abbreviated versions to the process.

Chaplains agree that amputees should be given the chance to continue serving in some capacity in the military after their recoveries. Those in the ministry who have been deployed more than once have seen the benefits of such decisions. They believe that a very important message is sent to wounded warriors when they are allowed to continue military service: they are valued, their family is valued, and their story is valued. Prior to such decisions being made, a different message was heard. Soldiers felt that anyone was expendable and their stories were demoralizing, regardless of the sacrifices made for serving one's country. This only intensified the flames of anger and resentment. Humans derive meaning in the commitments made to self and others. That thread of connection is simple, but powerful.

Successes

- *Pastoral support.* Additional staff support provided the necessary environment for chaplains to spend more quality and quantity time with wounded warriors at LRMC. It takes time to gain trust. Getting soldiers to talk about what they have been through is the first essential step in the healing process. Some find comfort in their respective faith, whereas others benefit just by having a caring person nearby who is willing to listen. Pastoral support extends beyond the bedside. Families also greatly benefit from counseling and comfort offered by chaplains, particularly if they have come to LRMC to say goodbye to their beloved solider. The medical staff also draws strength from pastoral support, and many look to chaplains for help when stress is particularly high. It is extremely difficult to watch patients die, especially after caring for them and watching them suffer. Chaplains play a vital role in addressing the emotional needs of care providers, as well as patients.

- *Chaplain day trips.* Fun is not usually the first word that comes to mind when one thinks of war or time spent at a military hospital. But fun is exactly the word that is used over and over every Tuesday, Thursday, and Saturday, when chaplains take outpatient wounded warriors on trips in the local area to help them relax and sightsee. Private donations fund these outings, and transportation and meals are covered. Soldiers must sign up for the trips and alert their LNO (Liaison Noncommissioned Officer) as to where they will be. They generally work the trips in between their medical appointments. The chaplain organizes visits to historical sites, scenic views, and tasty restaurants with plenty of ambience. Soldiers are permitted to dress out of uniform, and jeans, sweats, and sneakers are the clothes of choice. Volunteers supply cold drinks and snacks on the bus. It does not take long to hear conversation and laughter coming from behind the bus driver. Soldiers are able to experience the beauty of German architecture and the countryside. Trips during the month of December make stops at some of the festive Christmas markets, a German tradition. It is not uncommon to see American soldiers tasting bratwurst links cooked over the open pits or picking out a special Christmas gift for a spouse. Limb injuries, even casts, do not preclude chaplain day trips; wheelchairs get loaded on the bus and soldiers get wheeled around by a willing comrade with two empty hands. The value of these trips cannot be underestimated, for they repeatedly have helped soldiers restore a sense of normalcy and life balance. Chaplains have found that many are more willing to open up and talk after such excursions. Soldiers have said these trips give them a renewed feeling of hope and reconnection to the world outside of a battlefield. It is a day where wounded warriors feel valued and appreciated for the selfless service they have given their country. The trips are opportunities for soldiers to be with fellow comrades and "tell their stories." It helps break up their time. The positive impact had been enormous, and chaplains agree that it is one of the most effective components of their ministry at LRMC.

- *Care of the caregivers.* Although stress and burnout are common challenges during war, the implementation of certain routines helped to offset that reality. Universally, the chaplain staff will state that caregivers (including themselves), like wounded warriors, consistently need a safe and supportive place to tell their stories. They need to be reminded of the good they do all day, every day, and of the personal meaning derived from their work. For some, these types of conversations are most beneficial as a one-to-one conversation. Others have greatly benefited from the weekly Bible study groups started by the chaplain ministry. Hearing and seeing that each of them as caregivers are not alone with their feelings of grief, fatigue, anger, and frustration has helped with both healing and coping. Chaplains see that such support has attenuated a jaded and cynical outlook that is often prevalent in high stress work areas. Instead, most caretakers leave LRMC tired, but proud of their commitment and the outstanding care they provided. Other successful strategies have included family outings and marriage retreats. Addressing the needs of both couples and family is essential in maintaining the wholeness of couples and family units.
- *Volunteer programs.* See the "Chaplain's Closet" and the "Quilts of Valor Foundation."

Challenges

- *Reintegration.* More resources and attention need to be invested to help soldiers and caretakers reintegrate after their time of service when they return home. Family life is particularly vulnerable because this is an adjustment period for everyone. Spouses at the home front have been alone and working to keep the family unit going during deployment. They are looking to have their husband/wife return and resume their role as a shared partner. They often do not understand what their deployed spouse has seen or been through, many of whom return suffering from posttraumatic stress disorder. Soldiers and caretakers often find it difficult to talk about their feelings, or what they experienced during deployment. In a matter of days, a frontline Marine, for example, goes from looking at people and deciding whether to shoot them, to being with his fellow Americans in the general public. Each spouse has his or her own needs that get shortchanged and misunderstood at a time when each needs the other more than ever.

  Counseling is often necessary to help the family readjust to each other and to new roles. Both spouses have lived independently like a single person. They have each gotten into a routine that had not included the other. Although they love their spouse, it is hard to all of a sudden be a couple again. What is necessary for the day-to-day functioning in a military unit does not necessarily translate to family life. Soldiers are use to a set regime, doing what needs to be done to get the job done. For example, a deployed soldier might have been use to giving orders all day. This obviously would not make for a peaceful and happy marriage or parenting style. Simple tasks—such as driving, sharing meals, and scheduling their life with their spouse—are all part of the transition and require patience for all involved.

The divorce rate is particularly problematic, especially if there have been multiple deployments. An informal study conducted by the Army in 2005 showed that soldiers and their significant others rated the loss of their relationship as the number one concern regarding deployment, even more so than death of injury.[6] Family solidarity remains the most essential support for each soldier and the military as a whole. It is therefore paramount to recognize and respond to the unique needs of the military couple and family unit.

- *Burnout and stress.* With great meaning often comes great intensity. The level of devastation and trauma seen by the staff at LRMC would overwhelm the strongest of characters. Joy and sadness continuously exchange turns as the palpable emotion of the moment. Chaplains, medical professionals, and administrative staff work long hours, sometimes round the clock, caring for the various needs of their fellow American soldiers. What they would all tell you is that they wish they could do more. They are greatly humbled by the strength and selflessness of those soldiers they meet and who have been entrusted in their care. Eventually though, the physical and emotional exhaustion takes a toll, particularly for those on repeat deployment. Posttraumatic stress disorder is common among caretakers and chaplains as well. Strong support is essential for all caretakers and staff—while they are at LRMC and when they return stateside.

On his first mobilization at LRMC, Chaplain Pettigrew worked with almost 3,000 patients; during his second, it was close to 4,000. He can recall many stories, multiple faces, and poignant moments. He can recall resounding themes of pain, bravery, and heroism. But what will resonate most deeply in his heart and in his memory are the gratitude and humility of the American soldiers, even in the midst of their own pain and separation from their unit and loved ones. He remembers a level of energy that could only be explained by experiencing such overwhelming humanity, and that inspired Chaplain

Pettigrew and all of the staff to keep going until they dropped. They did not know how to do it any other way, and this was based on what wounded warriors had already done.

Chaplain Pettigrew returned to his position as an academic advisor at Western Illinois University. Like the returning wounded warriors, he, too, found challenges in reintegrating. He had to readjust his mind frame to a world that did not understand or know the bravery, selfless service, and sacrifices of wounded warriors or the medical staff at LRMC. He had to acclimate back to a college campus with the everyday problems and priorities of a college environment.

It was all so normal, all so appropriate, but so relative. He was primarily working with 18- to 22-year-old students, naïve still to the realities of work and world. Most of the 18- to 22-year-olds he had counseled at LRMC had already experienced several lifetimes of reality. Although he greatly enjoys his work at Western, a piece of his heart still lingers in the 3 miles of hallways at LRMC, a place that forever changed Chaplain Ronald Pettigrew.

ACKNOWLEDGMENT

We wish to thank Chaplain Ronald Pettigrew for his assistance with this chapter.

REFERENCES

1. Defense Centers of Excellence for Psychological Health and Traumatic Brain Injury. No Ordinary Warrior: Your Chaplain is a Frontline Resource. http://www.realwarriors.net/active/treatment/chaplains.php. Accessed April 27, 2015.

2. Landstuhl Regional Medical Center Public Affairs Office. *Fact Sheet–Pastoral Division, Landstuhl Regional Medical Center.* Landstuhl, Germany: LRMC; June 2009.

3. US Army. Chaplain Basic Leadership Course. http://www.goarmy.com/chaplain/about/basic-officer-leader-course.html. Accessed April 27, 2015.

4. US Army Medical Department. Clinical Pastoral Education Program. http://www.ddeamc.amedd.army.mil/GME/InterResPrograms/ClinicalPastoralEducationResidency.aspx. Accessed April 27, 2015.

5. Kübler-Ross E, Byock I. *On Death and Dying: What the Dying Have to Teach Doctors, Nurses, Clergy and Their Own Families.* New York, NY: Macmillan; 1969.

6. Miles D. *Army divorce rates drop as marriage programs gain momentum.* American Forces Press Service. January 27, 2006. http://www.defense.gov/news/newsarticle.aspx?id=14501. Accessed April 27, 2015.

Saying Thank You . . . One Stitch at a Time
The Quilts of Valor Foundation

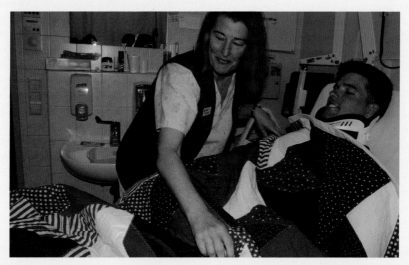

A Red Cross volunteer covers a patient with his new and very patriotic Quilt of Valor.
Photograph courtesy of the Public Affairs Office, Landstuhl Regional Medical Center.

It is a known fact that a mother's love can go a long way. A mother with a mission can go even farther. The Quilts of Valor Foundation (QOVF) started in a sewing room in Seaford, Delaware, home to Catherine Roberts. She believed that all returning soldiers should be welcomed home with warmth and appreciation for their service and sacrifices made for their country. After her own son's deployment to Iraq, she felt a need to reach out and give back to these soldiers. Catherine's sewing skills and the needle in her hand provided the answer. This desire grew into a national grassroots movement. Since November, 2003, the unique and heartfelt QOVF program has connected similar-minded quilters to wounded warriors and veterans.[1]

To date, QOVF chapters continue to pop up all over the country. Each week, groups meet at recreational centers, individual homes, churches, or any available donated space. Talented quilting volunteers are seen transporting their supplies to get the job done. The groups are often a mixture of every walk of life, age, and ethnicity: military wives, military mothers and grandmothers, their friends and families, and others with no connections at all to the military. The common thread is a love of quilting and a desire to volunteer and serve others who serve. One volunteer reports that quilt giving is a long-time American tradition dating back to the Civil War, when men going off to fight took a quilt from home, likely made with scraps from family members' clothing.[2] The American volunteer spirit has spread across the globe. Coalition members of the QOVF in the United Kingdom, Canada, and Australia are sewing patriotic patches for their own soldiers. The foundation has an impressive list of staff comparable to any business organization: a board of directors, regional and state coordinators, IT (information technology) manager, and coordinators for the newsletter, special events, distribution, membership, and many more. What is even more amazing is that all staff members are volunteers.

The communities of quilters stay connected through the very detailed and continuously updated website www.qovf.org. There is a link to the QOVF blog and Facebook page. The website provides instructions and *very* specific "do's" and "don'ts." Quilts range in size from a minimum of 55" x 65" to no larger than 72" x 90". Only high-quality 100% cotton quilting can be used. Softness is a must! In fact, quilters are told if they are unsure of any fabric, to close their eyes and rub it against their faces. If a fabric feels course, scratchy, or hard, it cannot be used.[1] Each quilt is bound, washed, labeled, and wrapped in a presentation case. Quilts of Valor are made to comfort and heal. The majority of quilters prefer using patriotic red, white, and blue colors. Stripes, stars, and every geometric shape and design imaginable are woven into unique and creative artistic blankets. Quilts are awarded at many different levels: individually, to military hospitals, to entire service units returning from deployment, and to the Department of Veterans Affairs.

Across the ocean, the impact of this effort is enormous. The majority of seriously injured wounded warriors arrive at Landstuhl Regional Medical Center (LRMC) with little more than the torn and blood-stained clothing they were wearing at the time of injury. Their stay may be only hours or days before they are stabilized for transport to a US military hospital for further care. The quilt is something personal and meaningful that is theirs alone. With so much loss that has often transpired in just a flash of time, this is something that stays with them.

Boxes of quilts arrive at LRMC from all parts of the country. Chaplains primarily distribute these blankets crafted with love. They are given to soldiers with wounds ranging from concussions, to blast injuries, to amputations. Nurses use them to cover their patients whenever possible. If the patient is hot or has a fever, they are placed over the footrest or at the bottom of the bed. Their beauty and brightness help offset the difficult moments when families see their loved one so injured or in pain. That splash of patriotic color goes a long way in humanizing the antiseptic smell of a hospital, endless walls of white, and a hospital bed.

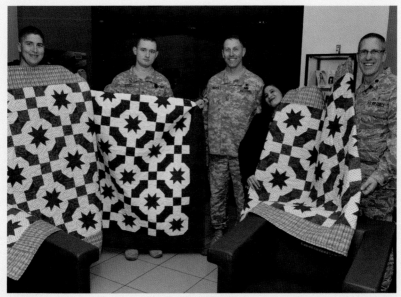

Soldiers display some Quilts of Valor.

Photograph courtesy of the Public Affairs Office, Landstuhl Regional Medical Center.

Quilts are given to soldiers who are awake and able to see and feel this gift, and to soldiers who are unconscious, intubated, and seemingly unaware. It is not unusual to see soldiers wrapped in their quilts while transported around the hospital in wheelchairs. Quilts of Valor have covered soldiers as they were being awarded with Purple Hearts, and they have covered soldiers while they were dying. No matter rank or circumstance, they were stitched with love and gratitude to convey a universal thank you from groups of quilters wishing to honor those who serve. Americans care about the comfort and well-being of US soldiers; their service, sacrifices, and valor are valued. Each quilt turns an ordinary moment of giving a gift into one that conveys a simple but powerful message.

To date, more than 110,000 quilts have been awarded to our soldiers and veterans.

REFERENCES
1. Quilts of Valor Foundation website. www.qovf.org. Accessed April 15, 2015.
2. NBC Nightly News. Quilts of Valor offer warmth to wounded soldiers [video]. October 21, 2013. http://www.nbcnews.com/video/nightly-news/53338284/#53338284. Accessed April 15, 2015.

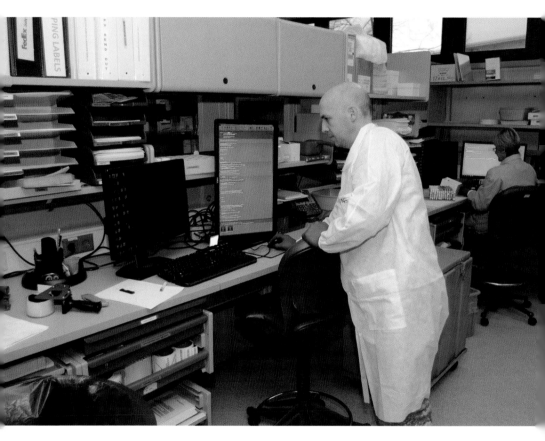

Laboratory personnel entering specimen information into
the computer at the counter designated as the "downrange
processing bench" at Landstuhl Regional Medical Center.

Photograph courtesy of the Public Affairs Office,
Landstuhl Regional Medical Center.

CHAPTER TEN

General Laboratory Services

*As the war progressed, clinical challenges at Landstuhl Regional Medical
Center brought about constant reassessment to improve patient care
outcomes and find optimum solutions through evidence-based best practice.*

L andstuhl Regional Medical Center (LRMC) played a pivotal role in
stabilizing and treating combat casualties for return to duty or for
evacuation to the continental United States for further medical evaluation
and care. Quality patient-focused care continued to be the highest priority amid
the constant changes and challenges brought to the hospital as a result of the global
war on terrorism. Each administrative and clinical arena continuously reevaluated
their respective services to meet the ongoing needs of sick and injured soldiers,
as well as the health needs of patients residing in the community. The primary
mission of the Department of Pathology and Area Laboratory Services at LRMC
is as follows: *To provide responsive, reliable, and high-quality laboratory testing in
support of patient care.*

BACKGROUND

Prior to 2003, the sole mission of laboratory services at LRMC was to
support daily hospital inpatient and outpatient laboratory needs. At that time,
there was no designated area to process samples from downrange because there
was clearly no need for it. This reality changed with the onset of the war in Iraq
in 2003, and then significantly again in 2007, when a troop surge of more than
20,000 soldiers was deployed in support of Operation Iraqi Freedom.[1] This
military strategy changed the patient care landscape thousands of miles away at
LRMC. Comparative hospital data from 2001 to 2007 showed that the average
daily census in the intensive care unit had tripled, and the level of acute care had
doubled. By November 2007, LRMC had treated more than 45,000 combat
patients with varying degrees of trauma from battle-related injuries.[2]

There was a significant trickle-down effect across continents as the complexity of medical and surgical care intensified for injured soldiers, and the impact at LRMC was felt hospital-wide. For example, laboratory services at downrange medical treatment facilities (MTFs) were historically limited to providing basic testing only. However, as downrange Role 3 hospitals increased their treatment capabilities, a greater variety of clinical laboratory tests were added to the standard menu to support routine healthcare, as well as the intense trauma care requirements. Versatility was mandatory in combat laboratories because the mission could change at a moment's notice. Downrange laboratory technicians could go from processing a basic chemistry panel, to typing and cross-matching blood samples from injured soldiers requiring immediate surgery, triaging the downrange hospital supply for available units of whole blood and platelets, or thawing units of fresh frozen plasma or cryoprecipitate.[3] Although the level of care had certainly increased, and downrange laboratories were handling several hundred samples per month, some of the necessary and more sophisticated testing could still not be supported. Deployed physician specialists were likely to order more varied and specialized blood tests that could not be done in combat facilities. Therefore, it became necessary for LRMC to become the referral laboratory for both Iraq and Afghanistan MTFs. By 2007, the laboratory at LMRC was experiencing a 25% workload increase; by 2009, it was at its highest workload capacity. Personnel were responsible for processing and testing incoming samples from downrange, as well as those from the inpatients and outpatients, who had also greatly increased in both volume and complexity of injuries.

Physical space was a precious commodity at LRMC, and there was not a lot of "extra" to meet the needs of various clinical departments and specialty services, all working at maximum capacity. The laboratory was no exception. Space had to be found in the crowded 10 by 25 square-foot processing area for the 30 to 40 boxes containing laboratory samples that arrived almost daily. All boxes had to be recycled and sent back downrange because they were difficult to come by in combat hospitals. Whereas the existing laboratory space did not permit any further expansion, a countertop was designated specifically as the downrange processing bench in 2009 because of the sharp increase of samples being received. At its peak, the bench was receiving and processing approximately 2,500 specimens a month from the Afghanistan and Iraqi theaters. Staffing adjustments were made to accommodate the operational requirements of the downrange bench, and two laboratory staff members were trained in CHCS (Composite Health Care System, a medical informatics system) and CoPath (laboratory software) computer programs. Every downrange sample (about 80–100/day) was hand-annotated that it was received, and then orders were manually entered into the computer for every requested laboratory test. Laboratory staff also adjusted to a variety of needs and tasks outside of the usual realm of duty. For example, large yellow buckets were used to hold surgical samples, such as fragments, any type of foreign body, heavy metals, and miscellaneous fragments for pathology analysis.

In 1994, the Armed Services Blood Bank Center, Europe, had been reorganized and moved to a facility on the LRMC campus. The chief of Blood Services was overseeing both the donor center operations and the hospital transfusion service. Blood Bank services became a more daunting challenge after 2003, when more and more critically ill trauma patients required multiple transfusions of various blood products as lifesaving treatment.

IMPLEMENTATION METHODS

After the surge, the laboratory department reorganized and consolidated all sections that handled any aspect of initial specimen collection or receipt. This included blood samples (phlebotomy services) and human tissue (department of pathology). The purpose of this new umbrella unit, now called Central Operations, was to ensure that only one section received, processed, and distributed all specimens coming into the laboratory from inpatient wards, outpatient services, and downrange theaters. Staff from Central Operations attended ward rounds daily during the week to assess the anticipated inpatient needs.

Funding was provided to hire additional personnel and to purchase necessary supplies and equipment needed to handle the extra workload. This was essential due to the high volume of patients within the hospital itself and to support downrange theater laboratory needs. Phlebotomy services also fell under the Department of Laboratory Services. Prior to 2003, there were four trained phlebotomists who collected blood for the outpatients at LRMC. Two more technicians were added to meet the increased needs.

The process for transferring laboratory samples from downrange to LRMC involved a great deal of organization and communication. This service gave downrange medical providers access to laboratory services and results not typically available in a combat zone. It also minimized unnecessary evacuations of medically stable soldiers who previously would have been sent to LRMC for laboratory tests; specimens could now be sent to LRMC rather than patients. The 5-step process was as follows:

1. Samples were collected at outlying theater clinics with laboratory facilities, logged in, and properly stored.
2. These samples were then transported to the nearest Role 3 hospital within theater. If that facility did not have the necessary laboratory equipment to handle the required testing, they were stored for shipment to LRMC.

3. The downrange Role 3 laboratory officer in charge then coordinated with the nearest Air Force transportation office, which determined the next available flight to Ramstein Air Base. Central Operations at LRMC's laboratory was also notified regarding the upcoming shipment.

4. Samples were then properly packaged and transferred to a CASF (Contingency Aeromedical Staging Facility) team for a MEDEVAC flight to Ramstein Air Base. These samples accompanied patients from theater transferring to LRMC for further medical care.

5. After arriving at LRMC, the CASF team delivered the samples to the hospital's noncommissioned officer-in-charge, who notified the laboratory for pick-up.

LESSONS LEARNED

The dedication and tireless effort of both the administrative and clinical personnel in the Department of Laboratory Services contributed greatly to the quality care provided to patients at LRMC. Successful changes occurred from valuable lessons learned as the war progressed, and the patient volume and needs intensified. Successes and challenges arose in every section of the laboratory.

Successes

- *Central operations: customer satisfaction.* All patients had an opportunity to submit customer comments either through an online computer program or a written card. The patient advocate office entered the results from received cards into the computer. Information obtained from submitted comments was reported at the laboratory's quality assurance/ performance improvement committee meetings and evaluated for any adverse patterns or trends. All dissatisfactory patient comments or complaints were thoroughly investigated and assessed for systemic problems and solutions. When requested, the laboratory also personally contacted the patient to discuss and address their concerns. The laboratory measured customer satisfaction monthly by percentage and posted these results in the patient waiting area. Staff wanted patients to know that quality customer service and patient satisfaction were taken seriously. The laboratory at LRMC served an average of 45,000 outpatients annually, and Central Operations consistently received a customer satisfaction score of 98%. The front desk staff, phlebotomists, and technicians who all interact directly with patients were consistently complimented on their attitude, professionalism, and expertise.

- *Downrange processing: transport of laboratory samples.* Between 2003 and 2009, laboratory samples were transported to LRMC from downrange

Blood Bank Services
New Initiative Brings Lesson Learned

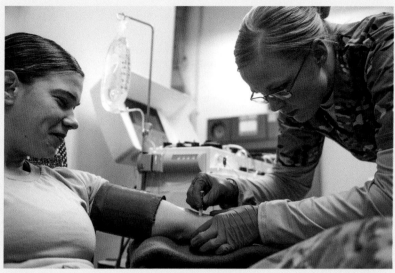

US Army Specialist Lauren O'Neal, 153rd Blood Support Detachment, medical laboratory technician, prepares to receive platelets from Army Specialist Samantha Criscio at Craig Joint Theater Hospital, Bagram Airfield, Afghanistan, December 31, 2015.

Photograph courtesy of the US Air Force. Photographer: Technical Sergeant Robert Cloys.

As the war progressed, clinical challenges at Landstuhl Regional Medical Center brought about constant reassessment to improve patient care outcomes and to find optimum solutions through evidence-based practice. Anemia is common in critically ill patients, particularly those admitted to the intensive care unit (ICU). The nature of injuries in combat casualties—such as amputations, internal organ trauma, and burns—often necessitated multiple blood product transfusions. The greater the length of stay in the ICU, the greater the likelihood the patient required additional red blood cell (RBC) transfusions.[1] Research has shown that the storage of RBCs over time leads to progressive degradation (known as "storage lesion") that affects RBC structure and function. Biochemical changes occur that decrease oxygen delivery to cells, and changes in the RBC shape increases the likelihood of occluding the microcirculation.[2] Adverse clinical outcomes in critically ill and trauma patients have been associated with these RBC changes, such as a decrease in tissue oxygenation and an increased risk for infection, multisystem organ failure, lengthened hospital and ICU stay, and mortality.[2]

The complexity of transfusing life-sustaining blood products was augmented by having to send samples from freshly donated blood for testing to the United States, where regulations are much stricter than those in Europe. No blood product could be released for use until test results were received. As a result of this requirement, there was an average lag time of 6 days from the time of blood donation to the time blood products were released to the shelf for use.[3] In 2011, the LRMC Department of Pathology (under Laboratory Services) and the Blood Services department identified an increase in the age of transfused RBCs used in ICU patients. Between May 2010 and February 2011, there were 941 units of RBCs transfused to 1,809 trauma patients admitted to the ICU, with a mean age of 28.5 days.[3]

Collaborative efforts then began with a multidisciplinary team comprised of trauma researchers, nurse educators, and pathology, blood service, and blood bank personnel. Several initiatives were implemented with the goal of reducing the age of blood in units used to transfuse ICU trauma patients. These included improving communication among providers, streamlining requests for blood products, and optimizing the blood bank inventory. One of the first policy changes required that trauma ICU patients receive packed RBCs less than 30 days from the time of collection. To further ensure that this requirement was met, a "newest blood" stamp was created for use on all blood product request forms (Form SF 518).[3]

The LRMC blood bank collaborated with the Blood Donor Center to improve response to blood product needs by scheduling and organizing area blood drives to maintain appropriate inventory. A designated "trauma shelf" was created specifically for storage of all blood products less than 30 days old. This improved identifying stock of the freshest blood units available and decreased storing older units of blood.[3]

Hospital leadership and the education department combined forces to incorporate training on blood product use and policies in general employee orientation. New clinical nurses attended hands-on training of the entire transfusion process, from collecting and labeling to documenting and administering blood products. A poster mock-up of the blood product request form highlighting the "newest blood" stamp was placed on all nursing units as both a guide and a reminder of the initiative.[3]

A blood utilization committee was formed to oversee and optimize blood product use at LRMC. This committee collaborated with the blood bank, the Pathology and Blood Services Department, the Blood Donor Center, and the LRMC education department to maintain all initiatives geared toward reducing the age of blood products administered to trauma patients.[3]

Finally, the Pathology and Blood Services Department worked with local and international shipping agencies to improve blood sample delivery and identification of the shipment to alert agencies of their priority status. This resulted in expedited delivery and a decrease in the turnaround time of laboratory results.[3]

A formal policy change was created at LRMC to reduce the maximum age of blood administered to trauma patients in the ICU from 30 days to 25 days. After implementing these various initiatives, data showed that the age of blood used in transfusions between March 2011 and December 2013 was 19.6 days, a 45% decrease. Additionally, the collaborative efforts of the Pathology and Blood Services Department and the shipping agencies reduced the lag time of blood product donation to the "trauma shelf" from 6 days to 3 days.[3]

Hard work, strong leadership, and collaborative efforts brought effective change. This evidence-based best practice was a valuable lesson learned that can be replicated in other facilities to improve patient outcomes when caring for critically ill and trauma patients in the ICU.

REFERENCES
1.   Corwin H, Surgenor S, Gettinger A. Transfusion practice in the critically ill. *Crit Care Med.* 2003;31(12):668-671.
2.   Vandromme M, McGwin G, Weinberg J. Blood transfusion in the critically ill: does storage age matter? *Scand J Trauma Resusc Emerg Med.* 2009;17(35).
3.   Chappell W. Age of blood: reducing the age of red blood cells and transfusion in critically ill and trauma patients. Best Practice Submission, Landstuhl Regional Medical Center. www.baylor.edu/graduate/mha/doc.php/228325. docx. Accessed August 16, 2015.

by means of commercial air carriers. This process proved to be highly unreliable because samples were not maintained in appropriate temperatures en route and arrived too late, no longer viable or stable for testing. It therefore became necessary to identify an alternative transport method. Successful coordination with the downrange processing staff at LRMC, medical personnel in the Afghanistan and Iraqi theaters, and the CASF team enabled specimens to be expeditiously shipped via MEDEVAC aircraft to Ramstein Air Base. This process was a success and reduced the average turnaround time for laboratory results from 12 days to less than 48 hours, and maintained specimen viability and stability. Once implemented, this important change allowed patients who were not seriously injured to be treated within the theaters of operation instead of having to be medically evacuated to LRMC.

- *Phlebotomy services: wait-time and quality of work.* The US Army Medical Command standard for patient waiting time requires no more than 15 minutes to elapse from the time the patient presents to the laboratory until served. At LRMC, the average patient waiting time in the laboratory was 5 minutes. The number of patient sample recollections was always consistently below the national average because very few errors were made by the labora-tory's well-trained and experienced staff. This was especially significant given the high volume of patients seen and the constant turnover of military staff.

Challenges

- *Staff turnover.* Personnel turnover continued to be the biggest challenge in the laboratory department. New staff had to be trained and brought up to speed in each of the various sections of the laboratory. This was particularly difficult when the hospital census was full, and sick and injured patients were arriving daily from downrange. In addition, the hospital remained 100% committed to continuing to serve the patients in the European community, so there was very little "downtime" in providing patient care.

  Turnover of providers in the combat hospitals was also a challenge for the lab at LRMC. The laboratory staff at LRMC entered the requested tests and provider information under the name of the person who sent and ordered the sample. However, that provider may have left by the time the sample was received at LRMC, and now staff had to spend time getting necessary information on the replacement provider to enter into the system. It was time-consuming for staff, and sometimes delayed running samples and reporting laboratory results to the care providers.

- *Communication.* Coordination was always a challenge with theater transportation units to ensure that the "right box of laboratory samples got on the right plane." Communication and organization were vital in this process, but errors did sometimes occur. As the war continued, lessons learned brought about changes and improvements to eliminate this from happening as much as possible.

ACKNOWLEDGMENTS

The authors thank Robert Hinkel and LTC Tracey Wilson.

REFERENCES

1. Abramowitz M, Wright R. Bush to add 21,500 troops in an effort to stabilize Iraq. *Washington Post.* January 11, 2007.
2. Fang R, Pruit V, Dorlac G, et al. Critical care at Landstuhl Regional Medical Center. *Crit Care Med.* 2008;36(7):S383–S387.
3. Sapasap S. Laboratory practices in a combat zone. *Lab Med.* 2008;39(8):453–457.

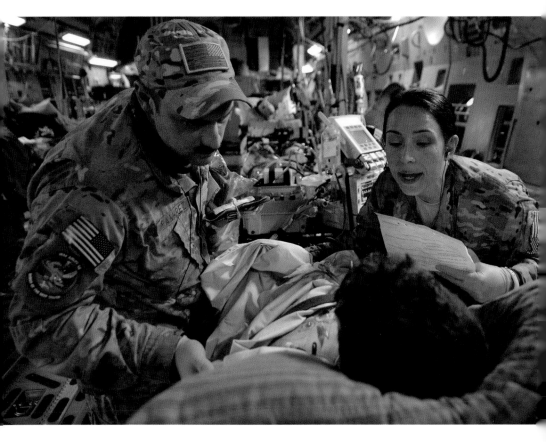

Captain Mario Ramirez and Captain Suzanne Morris, members of the 455th Expeditionary Aeromedical Evacuation Squadron Critical Care Air Transport Team (CCATT), confirm a patient's identity and prepare to administer a blood transfusion during a flight out of Bagram Airfield, Afghanistan, March 21, 2013. A CCATT crew consists of a physician, intensive care nurse, and a respiratory therapist, making it possible to move severely injured or gravely ill service members by air.

CHAPTER ELEVEN

Critical Care Air Transport Team

The Critical Care Air Transport Team is a highly specialized medical team that functions as a supplement to the primary aeromedical evacuation system.

The intensive care unit (ICU) in any hospital is a complicated, and often unpredictable, environment. This is the nature of caring for critically ill and injured patients. Now add factors such as noise from a roaring engine, vibration, dim lighting, fluctuating altitude, temperature extremes, and barometric changes of flight patterns. This is the reality of caring for critically ill and injured patients in the air, one of the most challenging care environments conceivable.

The Critical Care Air Transport Team (CCATT) is a highly specialized medical team that functions as a supplement to the primary aeromedical evacuation (AE) system. The concept behind its inception, in 1994, is to manage critically ill but stable patients who have undergone initial resuscitation in downrange medical facilities. Under the most challenging of physiological, psychological, and logistical circumstances, the CCATT has provided the highest level of care to complex patients with severe trauma, burns, respiratory failure, multiorgan failure, and other life-threatening complications. Across thousands of miles from Iraq or Afghanistan to Landstuhl Regional Medical Center (LRMC), highly trained medical professionals have monitored patients who are in a state of dynamic physiological flux and require continuous observation and intervention during transport to the next level of care.

BACKGROUND

Evacuating military casualties by air began during World War I, but it was during World War II that the US Army Air Corps organized an integrated AE system (AES). Nurses with specialized training in AE traveled with patients on cargo aircraft returning from downrange.[1] In 1942, the US Army Medical Service formed the 38th Medical Air Ambulance Squadron at Fort Benning, Georgia, and more than 1 million patients were evacuated during the last 3 years of the war using AE.[2] During World Wars I and II, however, it took weeks to months to move a patient from a combat hospital back to the United States. The average evacuation during the Vietnam War was 45 days.[3] Fast forward to the 1990s, when the AES had grown significantly and now included command and control functions, trained personnel, facilities for staging patients, and logistic support. Although this system was capable and successful in evacuating large numbers of *stable* patients, it lacked the capabilities to medically manage *critically ill* casualties.[3]

It became apparent that a reevaluation of the AES was crucial after Operation Desert Storm in 1991 and during United Nations peacemaking operations in Somalia in 1993, when the AES was unable to provide care for critically ill and injured patients.[4] The existing system relied on the transferring combat facility to provide supplies, equipment, and critical care specialists for AE, which then depleted their own capabilities to care for such patients at their field location.[1] The operational requirement identified a need to close the "care in the air" capability gap with a new program that would address the needs of caring for critically ill patients.[4] This need gave birth to the US CCATT program.

During the 1980s and early 1990s, Dr. Paul Carlton Jr (Air Force Surgeon General, 1999–2002) developed the capability to quickly and effectively stabilize critically ill patients for transport. He based his intervention on his experiences receiving casualties from the embassy bombing in Beirut, Lebanon, in 1983. In May 1994, Carlton and Dr. Joseph Farmer, a medical intensivist, launched the CCATT program, and a 2-year test phase was implemented at the US Air Force (USAF) medical centers in San Antonio, Texas, and Biloxi, Mississippi. CCATT's manning consisted of a three-person team, including a critical care physician, critical care nurse, and a respiratory therapist. A simulated critical care environment was developed, and each team was provided with the necessary supplies and equipment to care for patients during an evacuation flight. The physician on the flight was responsible for medical decisions if a patient's condition changed and warranted new interventions. The goal of the CCATT was to monitor critical patients and keep their condition stable without interrupting transport. After 2 years of pilot testing, the CCATT was formally approved and adopted into the USAF AES in June 1996.[1,4]

The initiation of the CCATT program occurred in parallel to changes made in military doctrine after the end of the Cold War. During the Cold War, large hospitals had been established in predictable locations in anticipation of large battles. These medical facilities were intended to hold numerous casualties who, if they could recover within 1 to 2 weeks, would remain there until their recovery was complete and they were ready to return to duty. Post-Cold War military operations, when the United States became involved in missions that were often unpredictable in timing and location, necessitated a different strategy. It was no longer feasible or efficient to set up large-capacity hospitals because locations of military operations could rapidly change. The goal then focused on deploying small but high-capability medical treatment facilities that would stabilize and then evacuate casualties as needed. Military leaders needed assurance that this strategy could safely evacuate critically ill and injured patients; the CCATT now ensured this commitment.[1]

IMPLEMENTATION METHODS

Organization

AE teams are composed of two to three nurses and four to seven technicians who provide care to noncritically injured patients and act as the liaison between the CCATT and the aircraft crew members. The CCATT augments the AE team through the capability of highly trained medical specialists who care for critically complex patients.[5,6] Each CCATT is comprised of a physician intensivist (anesthesiologist, emergency medicine specialist, surgeon, pulmonologist, or cardiologist), a critical care registered nurse, and a respiratory therapist.[1,4,5] Within USAF active duty, reserve, and National Guard units, there are approximately 250 CCATTs. Per guidelines, these highly trained professionals can transport three critically ill ventilated patients (eg, with extensive trauma or burns), six less acutely ill nonventilated patients, or a combination thereof.[7] The operational definition of a patient stable enough for AE includes a secured airway, controlled hemorrhage, and immobilized extremity fractures.[6] During Operation Enduring Freedom and Operation Iraqi Freedom, all critically ill and injured patients were flown out of theater to Germany by the CCATT.[5,8] The 10th Expeditionary Aeromedical Evacuation Flight, a deployed unit stationed at Ramstein Air Base, may fly several missions to Afghanistan and Iraq in 1 week to pick up critically ill wounded soldiers. They also then transport patients back to CONUS (continental United States). Often. these flights will be filled with different categories of wounded soldiers, the medical teams treating them en route, other passengers, and cargo. These CCATTs are primarily deployed from CONUS bases, though one team is part of the 86th Medical Squadron (MDS), also at Ramstein Air Base. The 86th MDS primarily provides AE capabilities for the European Command theater. The CCATT mission is only part of these teams' responsibilities; their primary duty is to provide patient care at LRMC.[9]

Training

The training for a CCATT is intense and highly specialized. Commanders nominate those USAF members with the skills and critical care experience to fill

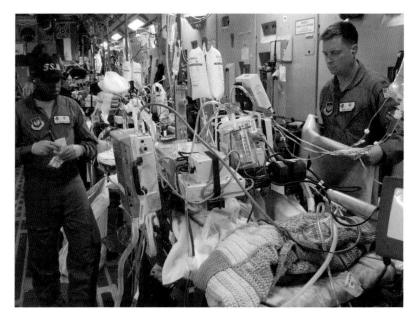

Air Force Staff Sergeant Napolean Gifford, left, respiratory technician for a critical care air transport team deployed to Ramstein Air Base, Germany, and Air Force 1st Lieutenant Brad Tiefel, the team's intensive care nurse, are part of an aeromedical evacuation capability that turns a C-17 Globemaster III into a flying intensive care unit as they transport patients to increasingly advanced levels of care.

Department of Defense photograph by Donna Miles. Reproduced from: http://archive.defense.gov/DODCMSShare/NewsStoryPhoto/2011-05/hrs_110505-D-5555M-005.JPG.

the positions needed to meet their unit's manning requirements. Each candidate must pass a flight physical. Candidates then undergo a process called *clinical validation,* whereby their training and experience are evaluated by a committee of CCATT crew members who serve in the same roles the candidates are applying for. If they pass this point, candidates attend a 2-week initial CCATT basic training course at the USAF School of Aerospace Medicine in San Antonio. This course covers everything from altitude and patient flight physiology to flight stresses, flight safety, surviving deployed environments, and equipment and supply allowances. Candidates are taught how to apply their critical care knowledge of caring for patients "in air" versus patients "on land." The AE crew also provides training to candidates in simulated aircraft cargo interiors.[1,4]

Teamwork is a vital component of the CCATT. The next step in training a new member involves participating in collaborative exercises that develop the vital teamwork required to interact and implement the multiple components of a fully deployed tactile AES. This training occurs during the Aeromedical Evacuation

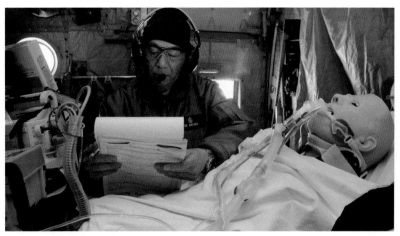

Lieutenant Colonel Ed Galvez, trauma nurse specialist, reviews HAL's medical chart during a Critical Care Air Transport Team exercise on board a C-130 Hercules. HAL is a male manikin-simulator used for training purposes.

US Air Force photograph by Technical Sergeant Bob Sommer. Reproduced from: http://www.minneapolis.afrc.af.mil/shared/media/photodb/photos/120205-F-TQ906-092.jpg.

Contingency Operations Training exercise at Sheppard Air Force Base, Texas. Here, candidates interact with other AE crew members, including those from command and control and ground staging facilities.[1,4]

Selected CCATT candidates then enter a sustainment phase in which they continually practice their clinical skills in their respective critical care area of expertise. When tasked for deployment, candidates begin CCATT Advanced, a 2-week course at the Center for Sustainment of Trauma and Readiness Skills (C-STARS) at the University of Cincinnati Medical Center, taught by both USAF and civilian faculty who provide intense training for military medical personnel in the areas of trauma and critical care. The University of Cincinnati was chosen as a C-STARS location due to its excellent reputation as a teaching hospital and its high volume of trauma and critical care patients. The C-STARS program provides the opportunity for CCATT members to refresh and enhance clinical skills and knowledge by working closely with expert civilian colleagues.[4] This course has three major goals for trainees:

1. review basic training from the initial CCATT basic course,
2. participate in 60 to 80 hours of critical care rotations in a busy Level I trauma center under the supervision of civilian and military faculty, and
3. incorporate lessons learned from ongoing operations at the civilian hospital into the training experience.[4]

This is the final validation process class for members, and evaluation consists of didactics, multiple real-life simulations, and a training flight using actual CCATT equipment, medications, and supplies. If the C-STARS faculty feels any candidate is not adequately prepared for mission success, that indivisual will not be deployed on a CCATT mission until he or she completes remediation training.[4]

Ongoing training is required to maintain current and updated CCATT skills. All CCATT members must reattend C-STARS every 24 months and maintain their respective readiness skills. In addition, all members must successfully complete a valid operational support flying class physical examination and possess a valid altitude chamber card.

Equipment

A combination of capability and practicality are the compromising factors used to determine the medications, supplies, and equipment carried by the CCATT.[4] Although the goal is to replicate the critical care capabilities of a hospital intensive care unit, there is also the reality of logistical limitations in an aircraft environment. All CCATT equipment is tested and must meet strict safety criteria. Standard critical care equipment—such as mechanical ventilators, physiological monitors, suction canisters, intravenous pumps, and blood analyzers—must be compact, portable, battery-operated, and flight-use certified.[1,4] The equipment must also interface with the aircraft oxygen and electrical systems, and be able to function amid constant vibration and temperature variability. A standard-sized canvas or nylon litter is mounted inside the aircraft, and metal brackets are strapped to poles that secure the patient to all the equipment.[1,4] All CCATTs are issued the same complete allowance standard weight of 790 pounds, which is packed in customized backpacks, specifically designated for CCATT. Between missions, the backpacks are designed to hang alongside the aircraft fuselage.[1,4]

The majority of CCATT missions are flown on the C-17 Globemaster and the C-130 Hercules aircrafts. The C-17 can support 36 litter patients and 54 ambulatory patients, whereas the C-130 carries a maximum of 74 litters. Only the C-17 has the capacity for on-board oxygen; portable oxygen tanks must be used on the C-130.[1,10]

CRITICAL CARE AIR TRANSPORT TEAM UTILIZATION
REQUEST AND FLIGHT PREPARATION

When the downrange critical care team identifies the need for CCATT transport, an AE liaison officer is contacted who then notifies a local flight surgeon to evaluate the patient and identify any special needs the patient may have in flight. The request is then forwarded to a Theater Patient Movement Requirement Center (TPMRC), which contacts the CCATT point of contact to discuss the

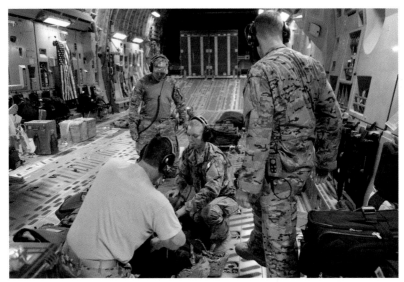

US airmen assigned to the 455th Expeditionary Aeromedical Evacuation Squadron (EAES) repack aeromedical evacuation (AE) equipment and supplies after an AE mission aboard a C-17 Globemaster III aircraft at Ramstein Air Base, Germany, August 9, 2015. The 455th EAES airmen are charged with the responsibility of evacuating the sick and wounded from Central Command to higher levels of medical care.

US Air Force photograph by Major Tony Wickman. Reproduced from: http://media.defense.gov/2015/Aug/20/2001274036/-1/-1/0/150809-F-LH521-154.JPG.

need for CCATT movement and to relay basic patient information. Once the request is cleared, an effort is coordinated with the Tanker Airlift Control Center (TACC) to locate an available aircraft for patient movement. An AE team, a CCATT, and the patient are then assigned to that aircraft and preparations are made for the flight.[5] The medical team from the sending facility turns over the care of the patient to the CCATT, who must be ready to accept the patient (often directly from the operating room) and assist in ground transport of that patient to the evacuation aircraft.

Careful and prudent measures are taken to prepare for this departure to ensure that necessary supplies are available and all equipment is functional. Prior to takeoff, preventive interventions—such as securing airway and endotracheal tubes, ensuring intravenous access, checking recent blood work and radiology reports, and reinforcing wound dressings—are taken to prevent in-flight crises. During this tenuous and critical period, the CCATT must be prepared to continue all interventions and resuscitation measures initiated by the forward facility. These include administration of blood products (packed red cells, fresh frozen plasma,

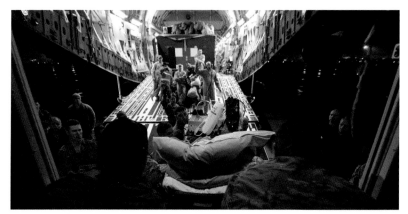

Members of the Contingency Aeromedical Staging Facility (CASF) and the 455th Expeditionary Aeromedical Evacuation Squadron Critical Care Air Transport Team assist patients onto the C-17 Globemaster III at Bagram Airfield, Afghanistan, March 21, 2013. The CASF is the relay between the Craig Joint Theater Hospital and aeromedical evacuation missions throughout Afghanistan.

US Air Force photograph by Senior Airman Chris Willis. Reproduced from: http://media.defense.gov/2013/Mar/28/2000063344/-1/-1/0/130323-F-LR266-081.JPG.

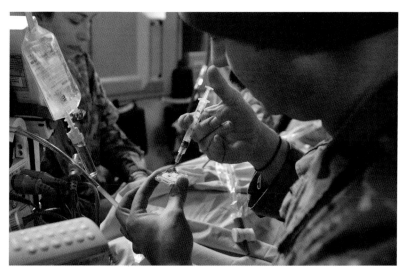

Senior Airman Delton McClary, 455th Expeditionary Aeromedical Evacuation Squadron Critical Care Air Transport Team respiratory therapist, performs an arterial blood-gas sampling during a flight out of Bagram Airfield, Afghanistan, March 21, 2013. The results will be used to monitor the patient's hemoglobin and electrolyte levels and guide further resuscitation during the flight.

US Air Force photograph by Senior Airman Chris Willis. Reproduced from: http://media.defense.gov/2013/Mar/28/2000063338/-1/-1/0/130323-F-LR266-136.JPG.

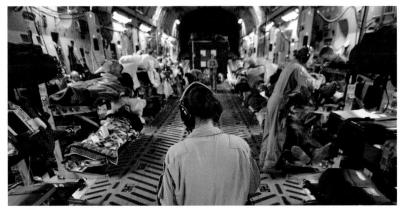

Members of the 455th Expeditionary Aeromedical Evacuation Squadron assist patients on a C-17 Globemaster III medical transport flight out of Bagram Airfield, Afghanistan, March 21, 2013. With help from the Critical Care Air Transport Team, the crew can turn a regular medical transport aircraft into a flying intensive care unit, making it possible to move severely injured or gravely ill service members by air.

US Air Force photograph by Senior Airman Chris Willis. Reproduced from: http://media.defense.gov/2013/Mar/28/2000063328/-1/-1/0/130323-F-LR266-222.JPG.

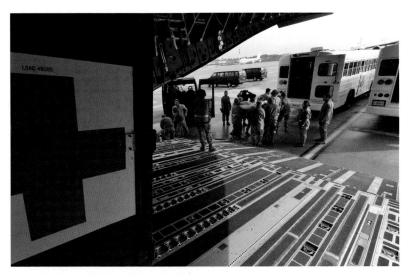

Members of the 455th Expeditionary Aeromedical Evacuation Squadron and the Contingency Aeromedical Staging Facility at Ramstein Air Base assist patients on a bus bound for Landstuhl Regional Medical Center (LRMC), Germany, March 22, 2013. LRMC provides state-of-the-art care using sophisticated invasive/noninvasive medical equipment and is the only tertiary intensive care unit within the European theater.

US Air Force photograph by Senior Airman Chris Willis. Reproduced from: http://media.defense.gov/2013/Mar/28/2000063325/-1/-1/0/130323-F-LR266-228.JPG.

platelets, etc); observation of amputation complications; and monitoring of ventilatory and cardiac support, intracranial pressure, chest tubes, sutures, wound drains, and external fixators.[6] Medical complications that are manageable in a controlled hospital setting can become quite a different and lethal challenge at cruising altitudes.[11]

CRITICAL CARE AIR TRANSPORT TEAM COMMAND AND CONTROL (AT LANDSTUHL REGIONAL MEDICAL CENTER)

When the CCATT crew arrives at Ramstein Air Base, they remain with their patient while the litter is taken off the aircraft, assist with getting the litter onto the AMBUS (ambulance bus), and continue to monitor the patient on the 20-minute ride to LRMC, where they report to the receiving critical care team that will then take over. There have been many occasions when CCATTs have delivered critically burned patients from Iraq to LRMC, where they are met by another CCATT who has flown to Ramstein Air Base from the burn center in San Antonio to transport burn patients immediately to this facility.[7]

When a critically ill patient at LRMC needs transport to CONUS, the CCATT point of contact is notified, and the decision is then made on whether a mission can be launched with 86th CCATT assets. This decision is dependent on the condition of the patient, length of mission, and availability of aircraft and aircraft crew. Because all the 86th CCATT members are fulfilling their regular duties, the minimum time for an alert and launch of a CCATT is 4 hours. This allows for CCATT members to be relieved of their patient duties and prepare for the mission. If, for any reason, a CCATT mission cannot be launched, the patient will usually be transported by commercial air ambulance.

LESSONS LEARNED

In the 12 years of conflict in Iraq and Afghanistan, the military medical system has effectively evolved to meet the needs of wounded warriors. The CCATT mission has significantly contributed to this effort. The nature of current military warfare and the use of explosives have intensified the need for exceptional trauma skills, both "on ground" and "en route." Developments in both the immediate critical care attention in theater, and AE transport across thousands of miles to LRMC, have resulted in improvements in patient morbidity and mortality. Even in the most austere settings, the highest level of critical care was delivered in some of the most defining lessons learned in these wars. They are described below.

Successes
- *Patient outcomes.* Between 2001 and 2012, the USAF CCATT program transported more than 8,000 critically injured patients, with

an associated mortality rate of less than 1%. This is a testament to the caliber and commitment set forth by every team member. Under the most extreme circumstances, this unique mission delivered advanced critical care never seen in prior conflicts.[12]

- *Implications for civilian practice.* The CCATT serves as a useful and successful model for hospitals to utilize to augment care during natural and manmade disasters, or to transport critically ill patients to facilities hundreds of miles away. Retrospectively, the CCATT would have been effective during Hurricane Katrina in 2005 or the 2011 tsunami. The CCATTs were utilized during the 2010 Haiti earthquake and successfully transported patients from Port-au-Prince to south Florida.[12]
- *Other settings.* The CCATT program is flexible enough to respond across a wide spectrum of operations and has been successful in a variety of situations, including humanitarian and relief assistance, homeland defense, military missions other than war, peacetime missions, special missions, and nation building.[13]

Challenges

- *Aircraft environment.* Even the most experienced critical care specialists would find en route patient care extremely challenging when compared to a hospital ICU setting. Although most clinicians are use to a certain level of noise, distraction, and fast pace in a civilian ICU, the austere conditions in an aircraft add a whole new dimension of challenge to delivering patient care.
- *Light.* The majority of CCATT missions occur at night, and light restrictions are enforced to avoid alerting the enemy. Clinicians must adjust to patient care under dim and minimal lighting, far different from a brightly lit US hospital setting. Routine clinical assessment of patient status—such as skin color (circulation), intravenous line patency, and interpretation of the color of fluid and wound drainage—is much more difficult and can be compromised in a darker setting.[6]
- *Noise.* Auditory cues (eg, as monitor and machine alerts and alarms), as well as normal conversation, compete against an average ambient noise level of about 85 dB inside the aircraft. Hearing protection is mandatory for all crew members, making questions and communication about patients' conditions or needed changes challenging and limited at all times.[6]
- *Vibration.* Both the crew members and patients are exposed to the turbulent and rapid ascent and descent of the aircraft (a tactical maneuver that is necessary for safety). The noise and sensation are additional factors

that contribute to the challenging environment. Acceleration changes associated with steep combat takeoffs and landings may lead to increased intracranial pressure in patients with traumatic brain injury.[6]

- *Altitude.* The average aircraft altitude during AE is 8,000 feet and can sometimes reach as high as 10,000 feet. The impact of a hypobaric environment on critically ill patients, and especially those with soft-tissue trauma from explosive injuries, cannot be underestimated. The lower oxygen content in the air, as well as the tendency for gas within an enclosed space to expand, is problematic. The CCATT must constantly assess for complications involving the presence of air or gas in the lungs, cranial cavity, or eye sockets. The altitude must also be considered and appropriate adjustments made when air is used to inflate endotracheal tube cuffs, Foley catheter balloons, and other medical devices. The effect of a hypobaric environment on life-sustaining equipment, such as portable ventilators, is also a constant consideration.[6]

- *Duration.* A typical AE flight to transport patients in the United States averages between 45 minutes and 3 hours. An average CCATT mission from Afghanistan to Germany is 10 hours and can take longer if other circumstances arise. The team must think ahead in preparation for extenuating time and circumstances for up to 72 hours.[6]

- *Emotional stress.* The extraordinary physical and logistical circumstances of a CCATT mission take an emotional toll on caregivers. They must draw on deep personal strength, courage, and resiliency as they face constant stress and responsibility when caring for critically ill patients under conditions of limited resources, sleep deprivation, and separation from family and friends. The mission is immensely rewarding but often isolating, especially in the face of limited options or resources when confronted with an unpredicted situation. A high level of clinical skill and knowledge is required to be a part of this unique team, as well as a strong physical and psychological readiness.[11]

- *Staff.* Because of its highly specialized nature, it is a constant challenge to find and maintain a sufficient pool of service members throughout the USAF who are qualified for the CCATT mission. There is an even smaller pool of members to draw from at LRMC. The challenge there is that members must commit to volunteering additional work hours beyond their regular duty assignments at the hospital. It is also challenging to keep members current and updated on the knowledge base. Fortunately, there have always been some CCATT members who have multiple deployment experiences to help instruct the less experienced members.

ACKNOWLEDGMENTS

We thank Colonel Warren Dorlac, MD, former Medical Director, Trauma and Critical Care, Landstuhl Regional Medical Center, and Major M. Josef Mikeska, former Director of the Critical Care Air Transport Team.

REFERENCES

1. Beninati W, Meyer M, Carter T. The critical care air transport program. *Crit Care Med.* 2008;36(7):S370–S376.

2. Martin T. *Aeromedical Transportation: A Clinical Guide.* Burlington, VT: Ashgate Publishing Co; 2006.

3. Zonies D, Pamplin J, Fang R. U.S. military advanced critical care air transport. *Soc Crit Care Med.* April 2, 2015; Clinical Controversies.

4. Fang R, Allan P, Womble S, et al. Closing the "care in the air" capability gap for severe lung injury: the Landstuhl acute lung rescue team and extracorporeal lung support. *J Trauma.* 2011;71(1):S91–S97.

5. Norton D, Mason P, Johannigman J. Critical care. In: Savitsky E, Eastridge B, eds. *Combat Casualty Care: Lessons Learned from OEF and OIF.* Washington, DC: Office of The Surgeon General, Borden Institute; 2011: 639–715. Chap 13.

6. Johannigman J. Maintaining the continuum of en route care. *Crit Care Med.* 2008;36(7):S377–S382.

7. McNeil D, Pratt J. Combat casualty care in an Air Force theater hospital: perspectives of recently deployed cardiothoracic surgeons. *Sem Thorac Cardiovasc Surg.* 2008;20(1):78–84.

8. Johannigman JA. Critical care aeromedical teams (CCATT): then, now, and what's next. *J Trauma.* 2007;62(6 suppl):S35.

9. US Air Force. *Medical Operations.* Washington, DC: Office of the Secretary of the Air Force; June 21, 2012. Air Force Doctrine Document 4-02.

10. Guerdan B. United States Air Force Aeromedical Evacuation—a critical disaster response resource. *Am J Clin Med.* 2011;8(3):153–156.

11. Brewer T, Ryan-Wagner N. Critical care air transport team (CCATT) nurses' deployed experience. *Mil Med.* 2009;174(5):508–514.

12. Zonies D. Long-range critical care evacuation and reoperative surgery. *Surg Clin North Am.* 2012;92(4):925–937.

13. US Air Force, Wilford Hall Ambulatory Surgical Center, Office of Public Affairs. *Fact Sheet: Critical Care Air Transport Team.* Lackland AFB, TX: January 2012. http://mldc.whs.mil/public/docs/report/hb/USAF_CCATT-FactSheet_WilfordHallAmbulatorySurgicalCenter.pdf. Accessed September 3, 2015.

Acronyms and Abbreviations

A

AAFES: Army and Air Force Exchange Service

ACS: American College of Surgeons

admin: administrative

ADVAB: Armed Services Vocational Aptitude Battery

AE: aeromedical evacuation

AES: aeromedical evacuation system

AFRICOM: US Africa Command

AFW2: Air Force Wounded Warrior

AHLTA: Armed Forces Health Longitudinal Technology Application

ALARACT: All Army Activities

ALRT: Acute Lung Rescue Team

AMBUS: ambulance bus

ANAM: Automated Neuropsychological Assessment Metrics

ANEF: Academy of Nursing Education Fellow

AOIC: Assistant Officer in Charge

AOR: area of responsibility

ARDS: acute respiratory distress syndrome

B

BAMC: Brooke Army Medical Center

C

CAC: Common Access Card

CAC ID: Common Access Card identification

CAPT: Captain

CASF: Contingency Aeromedical Staging Facility

CCATT: Critical Care Air Transport Team

CDR: Commander

CENTCOM: US Central Command

CFC: Clinical Flight Coordination

CHAMPUS: Civilian Health and Medical Program of the Uniformed Services

CHCS: Composite Health Care System

CM: Case Management

CMSgt: Chief Master Sergeant

COL: Colonel

CONUS: continental United States

CONV: conventional ventilation

COT: Committee on Trauma

CPE: Clinical Pastoral Education

CPT: Captain

CT: computed tomography/computerized tomography

C-STARS: Center for the Sustainment of Trauma and Readiness Skills

Cx: cancelled

D

DEERS: Defense Enrollment and Eligibility Reporting System

DFAS: Defense Finance and Accounting Services

DoD: Department of Defense

DRK: Deutsches Rotes Kreuz (or German Red Cross)

DSO: Deutsche Stiftung Organtransplantation

DV: distinguished visitor

DVBIC: Defense and Veterans Brain Injury Center

DVT: deep vein thrombus

DWMMC: Deployed Warrior Medical Management Center

Dx: diagnosis

E

EAES: Expeditionary Aeromedical Evacuation
  Squadron

ECLS: extracorporeal life support

ECMO: extracorporeal membrane oxygenation

ED: emergency department

ERMC: Europe Regional Medical Command

EUCOM: US European Command

eval: evaluation

F

FiO$_2$: fraction of inspired oxygen

1SG: First Sergeant

FMF: Fleet Marine Forces

FY: Fiscal Year

G

GME: graduate medical education

GSW: gunshot wound

GWOT: global war on terrorism

H

HFPV: high-frequency percussive ventilation

HIPAA: Health Insurance Portability and
  Accountability Act

HMC: Chief Hospital Corpsman

HMCS (SW): Senior Chief Hospital Corpsman
  (Surface Warfare Specialist)

HMF (FMF): Hospital Corpsman (Fleet Marine
  Forces)

HML: Helicopter Marine, Light

HMMWV: High Mobility Multipurpose
  Wheeled Vehicle (or "Humvee")

I

ICD-9-CM: *International Classification of
  Diseases, 9th Revision, Clinical Modification*

ICD-10-CM: *International Classification of
  Diseases, 10th Revision, Clinical Modification*

ICU: intensive care unit

ID: identification

IDF: indirect fire

IED: improvised explosive device

ImPACT: Immediate Post-Concussion
  Assessment and Cognitive Testing

ISS: Injury Severity Score

J

JPTA: Joint Patient Tracking Application

JTTR: Joint Theater Trauma Registry

JTTS: Joint Theater Trauma System

L

LNO: Liaison Noncommissioned Officer;
  Liaison Officer

LPN: Licensed Practical Nurse

LRMC: Landstuhl Regional Medical Center

LT: Lieutenant

LTC/Lt Col: Lieutenant Colonel

M

M&O: Movement and Orders

MACE: Military Acute Concussion Evaluation

MAJ: Major

MC: Medical Corps

MC4: Medical Communications for Combat
  Casualty Care program

MDS: Medical Squadron (US Air Force)

MEDEVAC: medical evacuation

med/surg: medical/surgical

MGMT: management

MRI: magnetic resonance imaging

MSgt: Master Sergeant

mTBI: mild traumatic brain injury

MTD: Medical Transient Detachment

MTF: medical treatment facility

N

NCM: nurse case manager

NCO: noncommissioned officer

NCOIC: noncommissioned officer in charge

NEMU: Navy Expeditionary Medical Unit

NFL: National Football League

NNMC: National Naval Medical Center

NORTHCOM: US Northern Command

O

OCO: Overseas Contingency Operations

ODS/ODS: Operation Desert Shield/
  Operation Desert Storm

OEF: Operation Enduring Freedom

OIF: Operation Iraqi Freedom

OND: Operation New Dawn

OPTEMPO: operational tempo

OTSG: Office of The Surgeon General

P

PAC: pay and allowance continuation

PACS: Picture Archiving and Communication System

PAD: Patient Administration Division

PADAE: Patient Administration Division Aeromedical Evacuation

PCV: pressure control ventilation

PE: pulmonary embolism

PERSCO: Personnel Support for Contingency Operations

PFC: Private First Class

PI: performance improvement

PIPS: performance improvement and patient safety

PMR: patient movement request/patient medical record

PTSD: posttraumatic stress disorder

PX: Post Exchange

Q

QOVF: Quilts of Valor Foundation

R

RAPIDS: Real-Time Automated Personnel Identification System

RBC: red blood cell

RN: registered nurse

RPG: rocket-propelled grenade

RTD: return to duty

Rx: prescription

S

1SG: First Sergeant

SF: standard form

SFAC: Soldier and Family Assistance Center

SFC: Sergeant First Class

SGT: Sergeant

SIPRNET: Secret Internet Protocol Router Network

SM: service member

SMEED: Special Medical Emergency Evacuation Device

SMSgt: Senior Master Sergeant

SNOIC: Senior Noncommissioned Officer in Charge

SOP: standard operating procedure

SSG: Staff Sergeant

SSN: social security number

stab: stabilization

STARTC: Soldier Transfer and Regulating Tracking Center

SVS: Society for Vascular Surgery

T

TACC: Tanker Airlift Control Center

TBI: traumatic brain injury

TBSA: total body surface area

TCC: transfer to continued care

TDA: Table of Distribution and Allowances

TMDS: Theater Medical Data Store

TPM: trauma program manager

TPMRC: Theater Patient Movement Requirement Center

TRAC2ES: TRANSCOM Regulating and Command & Control Evacuation System

TRANSCOM: Transportation Command

TSC: Theater Sustainment Command

TX: transport

U

USAREUR: United States Army Europe

USN: United States Navy

USO: United Service Organization

V

VBIED: vehicle-borne improvised explosive device

VIP: very important person

VTC: video teleconference

W

WIA: Wounded in Action

WTAR: Wechsler Test of Adult Reading

WTU: Warrior Transition Unit

WW: Wounded Warrior

Index